TEACHING QUALITATIVE RESEARCH

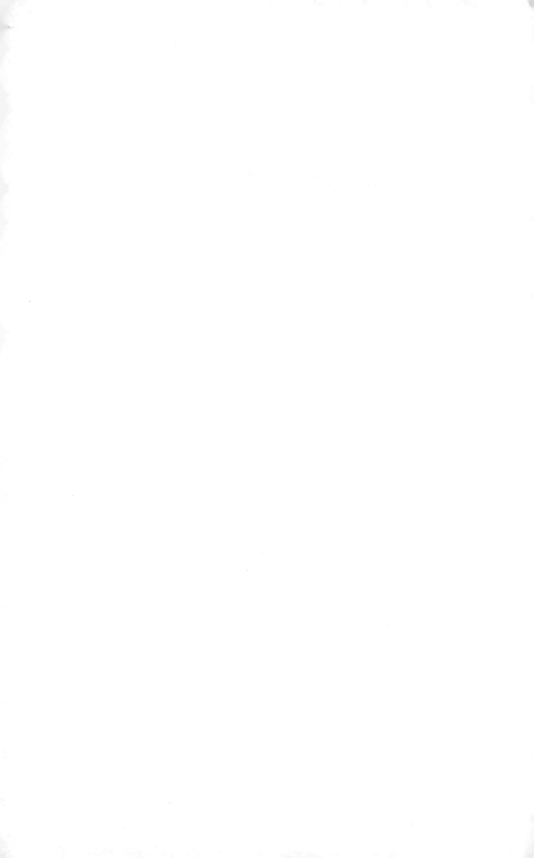

TEACHING QUALITATIVE RESEARCH

STRATEGIES FOR ENGAGING EMERGING SCHOLARS

Raji Swaminathan
Thalia M. Mulvihill

THE GUILFORD PRESS
New York   London

Copyright © 2018 The Guilford Press
A Division of Guilford Publications, Inc.
370 Seventh Avenue, Suite 1200, New York, NY 10001
www.guilford.com

Printed in the United States of America

This book is printed on acid-free paper.

Last digit is print number: 9 8 7 6 5 4 3 2 1

Library of Congress Cataloging-in-Publication Data is available
from the publisher.

ISBN 978-1-4625-3670-2 (paperback)
ISBN 978-1-4625-3671-9 (hardcover)

Preface

In the last decade, qualitative research has grown in complexity. Teachers of qualitative research play an important role in framing dialogues around methodology and socializing students. While texts on qualitative research are plentiful, they tend to focus on procedures, theories, and philosophies, leaving the pedagogy of qualitative research relatively untouched.

Teaching qualitative research goes beyond teaching content or techniques—it involves socializing graduate and doctoral students into ways of thinking and learning, to teach against the grain, to question assumptions and values, to pay attention to invisibilities and omissions, and to understand what it means to work within different frameworks. It also means being aware of the goals or purposes of research—whether it is a social change or social justice goal, or emphasis on perspectives that are overlooked or ignored.

This book comes at a time when the field has expanded in terms of approaches to and types of qualitative research, including tools for ways of conducting data collection and analyses. In this book, we draw on more than 40 years of our combined teaching experiences alongside a comprehensive review of the compelling literature. We offer content and exercises that can deepen the preparation of faculty into a community of practice, while building a more advanced pedagogical awareness and approach. Our aim is to make teaching research transparent and to infuse the process with a combination of curiosity, keen observation, and excitement. This book gives faculty teaching research methods courses access to a broad array of methods, paradigms, and contexts. It offers tools, exercises, and ideas for use in the classroom, and goes beyond a typical "how-to" book to illuminate the debates, discourses, and complexities inherent in teaching research.

We explore the difficulty of teaching students qualitative research at a time when quantitative pressures are high. We also discuss the pedagogical decisions that teachers of qualitative research have to make while thinking about their teaching. These include the planning of a course syllabus. We explain various course design processes and invite instructors to carefully consider what the pedagogical hallmark of the course will be and how to grapple with some essential questions when arranging the course. We draw on examples of qualitative syllabi to showcase the diversity of formats and the content in qualitative research courses. We then discuss what it means to think qualitatively and how to introduce qualitative thinking to students from the very first class. The chapters also cover teaching ideas and classroom activities to address a qualitative research project from start to finish.

Organization

The book's early chapters provide a foundation for the instructor, addressing teaching issues, approaches to teaching, pedagogical concerns, bias in qualitative research, and assessment in qualitative research. Chapters that follow address the arc of a research project, from conception to completion, including developing the research and ways to teach data collection, multidimensional approaches to teaching analyses, and writing up research for different audiences. There are activities and group work exercises in the chapters that can be used or adapted by the instructor. The book provides enough flexibility so that the chapters can be read in any order, to suit the needs of an instructor or particular class sessions.

Pedagogical Features

Taking seriously the pedagogies of qualitative research, this book offers the following resources for teaching that can be easily used or adapted and personalized by faculty for use in classes:

- Classroom activities for dialogue, brainstorming, and group work in qualitative research.
- Classroom activities adaptable for teaching research methods online.
- Classroom exercises for trying out qualitative research and for the practice of skills.

- Chapter overviews at the beginning of each chapter.
- Sample syllabi.
- Suggestions for further reading.

Audience

The purpose of this book is to speak directly to those seeking ways to teach qualitative inquiry within the social sciences, with special attention given to those within the various fields teaching qualitative inquiry as a means to preparing social justice-minded researchers. It can be used by faculty teaching qualitative research as new assistant college or university professors, instructors, or adjuncts; experienced teachers new to methods; methods teachers new to qualitative inquiry; and faculty who are trained and experienced in qualitative research. It can also be of use to those who are looking for materials and pedagogical strategies to assist students and emerging scholars.

Acknowledgments

No book is written by authors alone. There is usually a team that works to help with all aspects of the book to ensure that we are able to bring our best communication skills and style to the table. In our case, we have been extremely fortunate to have received the exquisite mentoring of C. Deborah Laughton as our editor. She has been with us every step of the way, always encouraging and supportive while also urging us to bring the best we have forward. C. Deborah has an unerring eye for the shape of a project and we are very grateful for the time she has spent with us.

In addition, we would like to thank Katherine Sommer, part of the production team at The Guilford Press, for her meticulous attention to detail. Along with C. Deborah, we would like to acknowledge the six anonymous reviewers, four of whom are no longer anonymous. A big thank you to Wendy G. Troxel, Director of Academic Advising, Kansas State University; Robin Jarrett, Family Studies, University of Illinois at Urbana–Champaign; Dorian L. McCoy, Educational Leadership, University of Tennessee; and Barbara Dennis, Educational Psychology, Indiana University, whose encouraging comments and careful, critical reading steered us in the right direction and helped us to focus the book.

We would also like to acknowledge all those who continue to inspire us in our journey in qualitative research, especially our current and former students at our respective universities, and our network of qualitative inquiry colleagues across the world. There are crossroads where we gather annually—such as the International Congress of Qualitative Inquiry, the American Educational Research Association, and the International Society for Educational Biography, where essential conversations occur—and the in-between times where technology keeps us connected and pushing forward.

Finally, we would like to acknowledge the power of friendship. Our friendship has sustained us over 30 years of research and writing collaborations—as well as navigating educational spaces as tenured professors within universities—that began when we were doctoral student colleagues at Syracuse University. We were welcomed into the qualitative inquiry "neighborhood" by trusted professors and given the skills and sensibilities we aim to pass on to others in the hope that they, too, will find the joy and satisfaction of creating new ways to understand people and the social worlds we inhabit.

Contents

CHAPTER 1

What Does It Mean to Teach Qualitative Research?

In this chapter, we lay out the map of the book and how we expect teachers of qualitative research to use it, and introduce the following topics:

- Why is it imperative that we build a pedagogical culture around preparing the next generation of qualitative researchers?
- What does it mean to "teach" qualitative research?
- The debates, discourses, and complexities inherent in teaching research.

Why Is It Imperative That We Build a Pedagogical Culture Around Preparing the Next Generation of Qualitative Researchers?

Qualitative researchers are socialized within departments by mentors and by the courses that they experience. They, in turn, go forth and disseminate similar ways of teaching. While qualitative research is dominated by books directed toward students who wish to start and complete a research project, over the last decade, building pedagogical cultures in qualitative research has become a central question. Researchers have begun to address, more and more, the issues surrounding pedagogies of qualitative research. The imperative to build a pedagogical culture around teaching research methods is based in part on the requirement for a qualitative research methods course, not only in graduate studies but increasingly in undergraduate programs as a way to build capacity in the workforce. Research methods skills are seen as transferable skills for employability, a point that is pertinent for graduate students, many of whom are equally likely to be employed by research centers, firms conducting market research, or by academic institutions. Building a pedagogical culture requires us to hold conversations and dialogues for an energetic interchange of ideas regarding how we teach and why we teach the way we teach.

The expanding scope of the diversity within qualitative methods makes it imperative that pedagogical cultures are made transparent rather than remaining implicit. In most course syllabi we have encountered, the mini field study remains one of the implicit pedagogical strategies employed, while others have looked at responsiveness or reflexivity as a key construct to build their syllabi around. A third way has been to focus on theory rather than procedure. Phillips (2006) has characterized these modes of teaching as the two poles, where one focuses on procedures and techniques and the other on ethics, beliefs, and values. There is, however, a large middle between these poles. The need for a bridge between the two poles is evidence of the need for multiple pedagogical cultures in the field of qualitative research. Our own teaching experiences have brought up questions from students that reflect both poles. On the one hand, we have encountered procedural questions from students, such as "How much data is enough?"; "How many people do I need to interview?"; "How many interviews do I need?"; "How many pages of transcription do I need?"; and "What is data saturation and when will I know I've reached it?" On the other hand, students have also asked questions about ethics and the politics of research, such as "How do I collaborate in the field when I know I will leave it soon?"; "Who am I to judge what the participants say?"; "How can I decide what claims I make from the data when I can choose from multiple claims?"; and "Should the participants analyze the data or should I?" Taken together, this book has been our attempt to contribute to a conversation about teaching qualitative research, even as we share what we have learned and continue to learn from teaching our students.

What Does It Mean to "Teach" Qualitative Research?

Teaching, as Waite (2014) says, is "messy" and "always unfinished" (p. 267). Teachers of qualitative research play an important role in framing dialogues around methodology and socializing students (Koro-Ljungberg, Yendol-Hoppey, Smith, & Hayes, 2009). While texts on qualitative research are plentiful, they tend to focus on procedures, theories, and philosophies, leaving the larger landscape of the pedagogies of qualitative research relatively untouched. Pedagogical questions about teaching research methods in general have been sparse. Wagner, Garner, and Kawulich (2011), as well as Earley (2014), reached similar conclusions that an identifiable pedagogy for teaching social science research methods in general has not materialized, yet a high need exists for its development. For example, Wagner et al. (2011) conducted a systematic review of 195 articles published in 61 journals from 1997 to 2007 and determined that a pedagogical culture for teaching research methods did not exist. By pedagogical culture they meant "the exchange of ideas within a climate of systematic debate, investigation, and evaluation surrounding all aspects of teaching and learning in the subject" (p. 1). A few years later, Kilburn, Nind, and Wiles (2014) extended this line of research by examining how faculty teaching research methods were breaking new ground as they moved forward toward a pedagogical culture. They examined 24 articles published from 2007 through 2013 (starting with 2007, the year Wagner et al., 2011, ceased their data collection) and focused specifically on "*how* teachers seek to facilitate the learning of research skills and capacities" (p. 192). Their analysis of this subset of the literature revealed that a new literature was emerging and on the rise in ways that support a growing interest in pedagogy. Drisko (2016) reiterated this point specifically for qualitative research methods and added, "we must teach each other how to be the best educators of qualitative researchers" (p. 304). Research skills are increasingly seen as a global asset that is transferable, increasing employability and creating an edge in global competitiveness (Nind, Kilburn, & Luff, 2015) with the pedagogy of research becoming an area of focus among researchers, employers, and funders alike.

There have been a few contributions to the literature that have provided important insights into the unique culture of teaching qualitative inquiry, such as Devault's (2010) chapter entitled "From the Seminar Room" in Luttrell's (2010) book where Devault interrogates and discusses the seminar she taught that helped her better understand the necessity and the power of reflexivity. We were doctoral student members of this very seminar and can attest to the seminal learning experience it was for all of us. Another innovative way to explore the complexities of teaching qualitative inquiry comes in Ellis's (2004) *The Ethnographic I: A Methodological Novel about Autoethnography,* where she examines autoethnography as a methodology through an account of teaching a graduate seminar on the subject.

Preissle and Roulston (2009) offered a chapter looking at trends and issues in teaching qualitative research and then Preissle followed up with deMarrais (2011) and used their years of collective experience to shape a chapter entitled, "Teaching Qualitative Research Responsively," in Denzin and Giardin's (2011) book. Hurworth (2008) made a different type of important contribution by interviewing faculty engaged in teaching qualitative research methods. Hurworth placed into the literature a productive list of variables related to the pedagogical challenges inherent within teaching methods courses. Furthermore, Hurworth claimed that a review of sample syllabi revealed little to no mention of the pedagogical approaches faculty intended to use, but rather simply provided topics. Eisenhart and Jurow (2011) added to the conversation by teasing out the various ways that research methods course objectives could be categorized epistemologically. Katz (2015), as part of a self-study of her own pedagogy related to her qualitative research methods course, sketched out some common practical questions often asked by those of us teaching qualitative inquiry courses: "Which chapters must be taught in QI [qualitative inquiry]? What should be their order? Should we teach one methodology in depth and others more superficially? Is it possible to change one's concepts about research in one semester (three months)?" (p. 353).

There also exists a growing area of literature related to faculty experiences with learning to teach research methods including some studies on a variety of social science research methods (Lewthwaite & Nind, 2016), qualitative inquiry in general (Abboud et al., 2017), or qualitative inquiry related to educational research in particular. As early as 2003, Creswell noted that faculty, in the area of mixed methods, were attempting to teach mixed-methods research courses at the same time they were learning their way through it themselves. Others have experimented with using the Scholarship of Teaching and Learning (SoTL) to collect and interpret empirical data related to their teaching. Crooks, Castleden, and Meerveld (2010), for example, conducted a SoTL study related to teaching research methods for the first time (within the field of human geography) where they identified some common challenges and how they addressed them (Crooks et al., 2010). Others have experimented with particular pedagogies, such as problem-based learning, for ways to teach research methods (Spronken-Smith, 2005) or archived/secondary data (Mulvihill & Swaminathan, 2019), or group-based assignments (DeLyser et al., 2013). Still others used forms of metaphorical learning, experiential learning, and collaborative learning processes (Mulvihill, Swaminathan, & Bailey, 2015). In another interesting case, Lewthwaite and Nind (2016), two scholars from the United Kingdom, convened an expert panel of international scholars to discuss teaching quantitative, qualitative, and mixed-research methods. They discovered that this group of faculty recognized that part of their pedagogical approach was rooted in their own experiences as doctoral students being taught and mentored by others. Another commonality was the bent toward activity-driven course designs that put students in touch with real data (either data they collected or were exposed to) in order to have the experience of trying to analyze the data.

Likewise, Kilburn et al. (2014) theorized that there are three dominant categories for research methods pedagogy—namely, active, experiential, and reflective. Some of the literature on qualitative pedagogy is centered on a critique of traditional delivery of methods courses. For example, Abboud et al. (2017) described resisting typical course structures by creating a pedagogical space that was student centered with faculty facilitation. They created an Advanced Qualitative Collective in order to have a space for co-teaching and co-learning qualitative research. By using the term *collective,* the group described and discussed a way to learn and teach qualitative research through pedagogical strategies that comprised a "Marxist approach to education, emphasizing collaboration, societal analyses and critical approaches to research" (p. 9). However, unlike most university requirements, the collective did not run a course per se and instead appeared to have formalized a fluid space that welcomed both doctoral students as well as advanced or novice researchers.

Scholarship related to teaching qualitative research methods in particular has historically been rare (Hurworth, 2008), yet a growing collection of resources have been developing (Breuer & Schreier, 2007; Cook & Gordon, 2004; Hammersley, 2004, 2012; Li & Seale, 2007) and the topic continues to be of concern to faculty teaching qualitative research. While the existing literature on teaching qualitative research methods is growing in sophistication, it is still scattered throughout various journals and other web-based resources. In addition, the content of the literature ranges widely in topics from discussions of course objectives to different disciplinary and interdisciplinary perspectives to teaching various types of students (i.e., undergraduate, graduate, doctoral) with various levels of prior research experience to actual pedagogical suggestions on a pragmatic level. The current state of the literature still requires those interested in learning how to teach qualitative methods courses and best practices for mentoring doctoral students to curate their own mini-library of resources from the scattered nature of the research, which may not feel as if it is speaking directly to their experiences. Pulling the literature together in a book alongside our own 40-plus years of combined teaching experiences has been a wonderfully exciting project for us and we are hopeful that others may find some benefit. Perhaps it may serve not only as a launch pad to help propel those preparing to teach qualitative research methods classes into the most useful and compelling literature but also serve to deepen the preparation by inviting faculty into a community of practice. We hope to assist faculty in building and sharing a more advanced pedagogical awareness and approaches that may help to further the discussion about preparing the next generations of qualitative researchers.

Some scholars have argued that teaching qualitative research and facilitating the learning process of students is challenging (O'Connor & O'Neill, 2004). Scholars have often pointed out the need to provide more transparent descriptions of the teaching activities faculty must engage in while teaching qualitative research methods (Koro-Llungberg et al., 2009; Luttrell, 2000). While instructors would like to improve their pedagogy, not much progress has been made with regard to determining what traits an effective instructor of methods would have (Wagner et al., 2011), nor do we know much about learning goals or assessment plans of methods courses and how they can contribute to student engagement (Howard & Brady, 2015). Our aim with this book is to contribute to making the mind-set and the associated acts of teaching research methods transparent, and to infuse the process with a combination of curiosity, keen observation, and excitement. A book on teaching qualitative research might easily look like another "how-to" book on qualitative research. While we intend to offer tools, exercises, and ideas for use in the classroom, our intent in writing this book is to go beyond a typical how-to book to illuminate the debates, discourses, and complexities inherent in teaching research.

Teaching qualitative research methods critically goes beyond teaching content or techniques—it involves socializing graduate and doctoral students into ways of thinking and learning, to teach against the grain, question assumptions and values, pay attention to invisibilities and omissions, and understand what it means to work within different frameworks. It means being aware of the goals or purposes of research—whether it is social change or social justice goals or an emphasis on perspectives that are overlooked or ignored. In this sense, we are responding to calls for research methods that promote social justice, inclusion, and empowerment of people (e.g., see Carspecken & Apple, 1992; Georgieu & Carspecken, 2002; McNicoll, 2014; Steinberg & Cannella, 2012). The role of an instructor in any classroom is to create space for student learning and understanding. These include structuring opportunities for students to learn from peers and to debate, discuss, and develop thinking skills. For teaching qualitative research, we put reflexivity and reflective thinking at the center of our pedagogical thinking.

To us, the essence of qualitative research is the search for meaning and the multiple meanings that are constructed in relationship. Whether it is in observing an activity, a place, or a group, meaning is constructed through the relationship between people and the researcher. In the interviewing process, or in creating and examining visual images, it is a similar co-construction. The researcher's positionality and relationship with the images, with what is seen and heard, and the looking and searching for the meaning of what participants reveal is fundamental to qualitative research—we relate this core idea to the pedagogy of qualitative research. Just as relationships and meaning matter to qualitative researchers, as faculty teaching qualitative research who are also socializing novice researchers, a holistic approach to qualitative pedagogy can keep the skills and spirit of qualitative research connected and integrated. In teaching, then, we do not approach skill building as separate from the emotional work that qualitative research involves and do not approach interviewing as a way to gather data, but rather to understand and learn from the participants what it means to live their lives. Context in teaching qualitative research can be seen as concentric circles with the classroom as the first circle. The context expands as we contextualize the teaching and learning of qualitative research to include multiple relevant contexts as graduate students carry with them the skills and spirit of what it means to question, be skeptical, and yet empathetic. Students can be doubtful and uncertain and yet confident with the ambiguity required to live within the questions, be skilled interviewers with compassion, and be advocates of justice and yet learn to tread softly where appropriate. These skills, attitudes, and dispositions are honed as the result of practice, deep reflection, and high-caliber mentoring.

Next, we present a review of the pedagogy of qualitative research by examining a range of articles scattered across several disciplines and subdisciplines, and published as refereed journal articles, book chapters, and online resources. We synthesize the work of scholars who have examined their own teaching and in some cases others' teaching of several aspects and dimensions of research methodologies and methods.

Introduction to the Debates, Discourses, and Complexities Inherent in Teaching Research

Teaching research involves several decisions that range from course design choices to figuring out ways to structure experiences that promote creativity and learning in students. Teaching research so that we centralize meaning making means engaging in pedagogical thinking at the intersection of clarity, complexity, and spontaneity. Teaching, like learning, is complex and multifaceted. Teaching qualitative research is inherently complex, requiring us to become cognizant of the debates, discourses, and issues inherent in teaching, and in particular, in teaching research.

Different Fields and the Issues in Common for Teaching Qualitative Research

Qualitative research over the last few decades has grown beyond the disciplines of anthropology, sociology, and education to embrace most social science disciplines (e.g., geography, urban studies) and disciplines of the professions (e.g., nursing, social work). DeLyser (2008) explains that one of the difficulties of teaching qualitative research is determining whether qualitative research courses need to be taught so that they are discipline specific or taught so that they cross disciplinary boundaries. Further challenges for faculty who teach qualitative courses for the first time is learning to figure out how to respond to the inexperience of students; make decisions regarding what to include or exclude in terms of course readings, focus, and fieldwork; and how to assess whether students learned what we intended them to learn in the course.

Teaching Qualitative Research in Quantitative Times

Teaching qualitative methods in an era of big data needs careful examination and unpacking. One of the challenges that faculty face when designing and teaching qualitative research courses includes the growing trend toward using "big data" quantitative studies that seem to dominate educational research policy-level discussions. Pressure to develop and train student researchers in quantitative skills may persist. Helping students to understand the relationship between their qualitative research skills and resulting studies and mixed-methods and quantitatively driven approaches will no doubt need to be part of the research methodological discussion. Thankfully, there are a number of helpful resources that can be used as guides. For example, Leavy's (2017) accessible and highly practical research design book *Research Design: Quantitative, Qualitative, Mixed Methods, Arts-Based, and Community-Based Participatory Research Approaches* and Creswell's (2018) *Research Design: Qualitative, Quantitative, and Mixed Methods Approaches, Fourth Edition* help novice researchers grasp the basic tenets of these approaches. And Johnson and Onwuegbuzie's (2004) often-cited article "Mixed Methods Research: A Research Paradigm

Whose Time Has Come," posits an argument for why it is a necessity for all researchers (including qualitative researchers) to have a clear understanding of mixed methods and their uses.

There is a rich diversity within qualitative research that can be used for teaching without teaching it as an alternative to quantitative data or in opposition to big data. Doing the latter might obscure the depth and multiplicity of choices that exist within qualitative research. In order to teach qualitative methods so that its diversity is drawn out, especially in the current era of big data, students must be exposed to a whole spectrum of research methodologies in order to more fully understand the strengths and limitations of each.

Institutional Arrangements and Politics

Waite (2014) identified what he referred to as "the (micro)politics at play within departments and programs" (p. 270) that can impact the experience of those teaching qualitative research methods courses. The particular departmental home for these courses, whether the courses are cross-listed with other departments; who is deemed qualified to teach the courses; whether the courses are designed as face-to-face, hybrid, workshop based, studio based, or online; and whether they are required or electives, all represent decisions that matter to those of us teaching the courses and to the students taking these courses. Several of these decisions are made without the input of the faculty but can impact the quality and content of the course. Face-to-face courses are performed differently and require different types of preparation on the part of faculty teaching the course than when teaching online or hybrid. Teaching performances are shaped by many things, including the delivery medium.

Charmaz (2015), for example, suggested that qualitative research course structures and content are largely dependent on departmental requirements, and a single course, or even two courses, are unlikely to fulfill the needs of students for analytical training and practice. Charmaz suggests that short, intensive courses and workshops in addition to regular research courses might succeed in teaching students analysis and in keeping the momentum of their research. In addition, Charmaz calls for creating a "cadre of qualitative methodologists" (p. 1619) who can draw on a variety of strategies to teach qualitative research, and in particular, qualitative theory construction and analysis. We offer various ways to think about the forms and functions of qualitative inquiry courses while recognizing that particular contexts and situations will require modifications.

CHAPTER SUMMARY ● ● ● ● ● ● ● ● ● ● ●

The key ideas shared in this chapter centered around our motivations for writing this book, including our argument for why is it imperative that we build a pedagogical culture around preparing the next generation of qualitative researchers and our interest in providing a practical resource for those who teach qualitative inquiry courses. In addition, we introduced the debates, discourses, and complexities inherent in teaching research. We hope this introductory chapter provided you with a foothold into the book and you will join us in the ensuing chapters as we explore the various layers of what constitutes a pedagogical culture for qualitative inquiry. Next, Chapter 2 tackles the pathways faculty find themselves on when they begin teaching qualitative inquiry courses and the attending socialization processes.

CHAPTER 2

So You've Been Asked to Teach a Qualitative Research Course

Socialization and the Qualitative Researcher

In this chapter, we use the existing research on teaching to point out that teachers often reflect their own socialization in their teaching. We argue that teaching qualitative research goes beyond teaching skills or content—it involves the socialization of students into the research process. We touch on the difficulty of teaching students qualitative research at a time when quantitative pressures are high and discuss the pedagogical decisions that teachers of qualitative research have to make while thinking about their teaching. We provide ways to design course syllabi and offer a few examples to showcase a variety of approaches taken. The first job that teachers of qualitative research have to undertake is to design a course and plan a course syllabus, although at times they are handed a syllabus used by a prior instructor and expected to use it. In this chapter, we address the conditions and decisions faculty often need to make when being assigned a qualitative research methods course to teach. Course design processes invite the teacher to carefully consider what the pedagogical hallmark of the course will be and forces the teacher to grapple with some essential questions while pragmatically arranging the course.

In short, this chapter focuses on:

- The process of designing a course, or modifying an existing course, that will serve as a blueprint for teaching a qualitative inquiry course.

- Course design principles, processes, and taxonomies as well as specific guidelines to assist faculty with building a course.

- The socialization process that takes place for novice researchers and how it impacts pedagogical decisions.
- Various approaches and delivery methods used to teach qualitative inquiry courses.

Course Design Principles, Processes, and Taxonomies

Bloom's (1956) *Taxonomy of Educational Objectives* and the subsequently revised and enhanced ideas surrounding his work, such as Marzano and Kendall (2006), are always useful starting points when contemplating course design. The taxonomy includes the following domains: knowledge, comprehension, application, analysis, synthesis, and evaluation. Considering learning objectives from each of these levels or domains helps course designers maintain an alignment between course objectives, assignments and activities, and pedagogical approaches, as well as assessment and evaluation approaches.

In addition to Bloom's (1956) taxonomy and Marzano and Kendall's (2006) revisions to Bloom's taxonomy, Fink (2003) has identified five principles meant to guide the development of high-impact pedagogical practices. These ideas collectively can be used to guide the types of learning central to qualitative inquiry courses. Three of the principles offered by Fink are concerned with how to teach (1) active learning; (2) challenging students to significant forms of learning; and (3) developing a system of feedback, assessment, and grading. Two other principles describe the qualities of a good teacher: (4) those who can develop good relationships with students; and (5) those who are caring about students, learning, teaching, and the content of what they have taught. Fink points out that teachers have traditionally used Bloom's taxonomy of cognitive learning to facilitate their teaching. However, there are skills and dispositions that do not fit the taxonomy easily and need to go beyond it—learning to adapt or change, learning how to learn, interpersonal skills, ethics or character, and communication skills. All of these imply a change taking place in the learner, a point Fink emphasized while creating a new taxonomy of what he called "significant learning," incorporating the following six dimensions: (1) foundational knowledge, (2) application, (3) integration, (4) human dimension, (5) caring, and (6) learning how to learn. An important feature of Fink's taxonomy is that learning is interactive but nonhierarchical.

Fink's (2003) point is that it is important for instructors to construct learning goals for a course that goes beyond mastering the content to finding a way to connect with the content and applying it to solving issues or understanding a problem. In other words, learning is not a singular act—it involves the mastery of multiple skills and dispositions as well as different types of knowledge (Fry, Kettridge, & Marshall, 2009; Sargeant, 2012). This would then lead learners to make their learning significant and worth pursuing so as to help them connect their learning to their lives. They would also keep learning independently, even after the end of the course, since they would care about the subject matter and its political or social implications. Fink urges instructors to be clear about the different types of thinking they want students to engage with in their courses. He offers Sternberg's (1989) three types of thinking as an illustration. The first is critical thinking that would involve analysis and evaluation, the second is creative thinking that would be imaginative, and the third is practical thinking that would require students to apply what they have learned to an issue or problem.

If we adapt Fink's (2003) guidelines and apply them to designing qualitative research methods courses, an example of what learning goals might look like follows. (Given our interest in making holistic approaches to education of paramount importance, we have added to Fink's taxonomy an aesthetic dimension, which includes learning to be attentive to emotions and one's own embodied responses as a learner and instructor. We offer this as an example that instructors can adapt as goals for their own courses.)

• *Learn foundational knowledge.* Here we could outline some aspects of what students could learn regarding the subject matter of qualitative research: learn the vocabulary of qualitative research; learn the basics of qualitative research and distinguish it from quantitative research; read critically and read studies in qualitative research; learn the basic features of qualitative research; and learn how to conduct qualitative research. Through this goal students would also learn critical thinking of analysis and evaluation.

• *Application.* This goal could be realized through an objective where students would apply the principles of qualitative research to conduct a small-scale study. To conduct a study students would need to read the literature and learn to distill information and synthesize the scholarly work, and learn to craft a qualitative question and apply it to a research problem or issue. Students would learn to craft qualitative research designs and learn the skills of gathering different types of qualitative data, manage and analyze the data, and learn to write the findings of their study. Skills could also include learning to present research in conference contexts, and learning to debate and discuss the different issues in qualitative research. In this goal, students would learn practical thinking—in other words, how to apply the principles of qualitative research to a study.

- *Integration.* Students would learn to see the interaction between different types of qualitative research and the different philosophies and assumptions underlying research. They would learn to find connections between the work of scholars, theories, and their own research purpose and would learn to synthesize and critique the literature. This goal would help students learn critical thinking and evaluation and analytical skills.

- *Human dimension.* Students will identify the ways in which qualitative research projects can affect participants and the researchers equally. They will also identify the ways in which research can benefit communities of practice and the field of scholarship. This goal would help students engage in creative thinking that is imaginative in addition to utilizing critical thinking skills.

- *Caring.* Students would learn the ethics of research and be mindful of the confidentiality and protection of participants and would approach participants with curiosity and respect. This goal would help students to think with their hearts as well as their minds as they bring the caring dimension into the forefront of their research practice.

- *Aesthetic dimension.* While the aesthetic dimension intersects with the human and caring attributes, it is also distinct in that the students learn to develop embodied awareness and be attentive to their emotions as they prepare and conduct research. This goal emphasizes self-awareness in the qualitative research process, and would help students to utilize artistic thinking where continuous appraisal and observation leads to an enhanced discernment and perception on the part of the researcher.

- *Learning how to learn.* Student researchers would practice reflexivity so that they are aware of their own learning in the context of their research. Students would also raise new questions for further research at the conclusion of their projects, which would allow them to engage in peer review and offer themselves and others constructive feedback.

Design Principles of Courses and Understanding the Learner

Sargeant (2012) describes and reflects on her assumptions regarding students' learning styles in a qualitative teaching experience. Her course design had plenty of activities built into it—however, such activities would probably appeal only to those students whose learning style matched taking on new activities and challenges with enthusiasm. She questioned her own assumption that the learning objectives, the activities, or teaching style and assessments that she designed would all be automatically aligned. Looking at Biggs's (1996) work, Sargeant began to pay attention to whether or not her course aligned and mapped these aspects effectively. She points out that in reflecting on her course, she realized that she had focused more on covering the subject matter rather than facilitating student learning. Norton (2009) cautions that while constructive alignment of assessment and learning outcomes is desirable, it should not become mechanical, thereby defeating the purpose—creating meaningful learning experiences for students.

Breadth or depth is one question regarding course design that instructors have to routinely make. This decision is also, in part, dependent on the curricular requirements of departments. There are also political considerations that at times need to be addressed or at least understood. For example, as Waite (2014) attests, "One issue here is whether anyone can teach qualitative research. At many universities, faculty are thought competent to teach qualitative research methods if they did a qualitative dissertation themselves. Absent are the questions of quality, of experience, of depth of understanding, even of pedagogical skill" (p. 278, fn. 5). Elton (2001) and Simons and Elen (2007) emphasize the need to go beyond a research record and consider pedagogical skills and teaching abilities on the part of faculty asked to teach research methods. Wagner et al. (2011) suggest that there is a need for research and debate regarding the teaching of research methods and what makes a successful research methods teacher.

Graduate school and completing a PhD does not always prepare one to teach in higher education. While the process of qualitative research might have become ingrained in one, it is often difficult to articulate the exact process that one followed, much less teach novice researchers how to research or answer the varied questions that are inseparable from the diverse topics that students in a qualitative course would like to pursue. And yet, it is fairly routine to ask new faculty to teach a research methods course. The natural default mode of teaching is to teach as one has been taught or as one has conducted one's own research. For example, faculty who have completed a case study for their own research are likely to focus on case study as the primary approach in qualitative research. Others might decide that theory should drive the research project and therefore emphasize theory, while still others might want their students to "get their feet wet" in the field and therefore focus on learning to take field notes. The decisions that one needs to make when being asked to teach qualitative research are many for new faculty—these can be fun, creative, and enjoyable instead of anxiety provoking. One way to begin to ease the anxiety is perhaps to move away from the emphasis on how to teach and instead consider what we might want students to learn and begin building the course from that foundation.

Beginning teachers of qualitative research may also be in the process of forging a teaching identity, trying to answer the question of Who am I when I am teaching? And in particular, What is my teaching identity when I teach research methods courses?; What type of teacher do I want to be?; and What do I value most in my classroom? These thoughts and questions are natural and are often revisited, even by those who have been teaching for several years. Research on university faculty emphasizes the point that their personal experiences as graduate students carry over into their own teaching approaches. To help disrupt an unexamined carryover of prior examples of teaching often requires intentional reexamination of one's teaching identity and to have room to grapple with the options that can be taken up. The ground level, however, needs to name the pedagogical theory or value system that will be used to guide the more pragmatic aspects of the work. In this book, we have worked to emphasize a critical framework and develop holistic pedagogical approaches as ways to teach qualitative research in order to name the value system surrounding our ideas.

Approaches to Teaching Qualitative Research

The issues within qualitative teaching may not be fully articulated (Wagner et al., 2011) since much of the reporting by those teaching qualitative research is scattered throughout several disciplinary journals. From the literature available on teaching qualitative research across disciplines, we can safely surmise that the discourse of teaching and learning in qualitative research methods is still in its infancy.

The following sections explore some questions that come up for both the philosophical and practical levels.

Should Qualitative Research Be Taught within Single Disciplines or Should a Cross-Disciplinary Approach Be Advocated?

Institutions have different responses to this question, some of which are determined by funding rather than driven by the need to evaluate the curricula or approaches to research methods teaching. Scholars have had mixed responses to this question and have argued vigorously on both sides of the debate. Some scholars have advocated cross-disciplinary teaching of qualitative research as being beneficial to students. Benefits include students having the opportunity to explore new research questions or being better prepared for cross-disciplinary collaboration (Preissle & Roulston, 2009; Simons & Elen, 2007). Other scholars (Lorenz, 2003; Welch & Panelli, 2003) argue that teaching research methods within disciplinary contexts is more effective. In the latter case, methods could be augmented with disciplinary content and presented in the context of disciplinary debates (Howard & Brady, 2015).

Why Teach Critically? What Other Approaches Are Possible?

Teaching from a critical framework, for us, does not exclude interpretive frameworks, nor does it exclude activity-based learning or culturally responsive pedagogies. Critical teaching draws from a holistic framework that embraces a variety of pedagogies and keeps reflexivity at its center. We draw from a holistic framework that is linked to our own experiences of holistic pedagogies in which attention to the relational aspect of learning is paramount. For us, our experiences in either teaching in holistic schools or having a passion for biography served as the foundation for an abiding interest in and deep investigation into holistic teaching. For faculty to teach from a critical approach means the opportunity to be reflective and learn from teaching. The vast choices available for teachers of qualitative research makes teaching an exciting endeavor, one that requires planning and thinking. O'Connor and O'Neill (2004) point out that one of the challenges of teaching qualitative research is figuring out ways to make students aware of their deeply embedded assumptions regarding research, and in addition, to counter a positivistic attitude of mind.

Teaching Face-to-Face

Teaching, for us, is a commitment to inquiry, creativity, and dialogue. These three dimensions of teaching are scaffolded by reflexivity as our own learning develops in parallel to our teaching practice. To us, teaching is holistic, a way by which we can examine assumptions, grow awareness, and treat dialogue and silence as equally significant in the creation of a classroom community. Teaching face-to-face is to challenge ourselves to communicate with immediacy, and bring our whole selves to the relational context of the higher-education classroom. However, the exercises that we offer in this book can be used for face-to-face teaching and can also be adapted for online pedagogy.

Teaching Online

Teaching qualitative research online can present unique challenges that might be similar to those faced by teachers of application-oriented subjects or topics. However, nursing, for example, has adapted to the online platform and found ways to teach practice that qualitative research can emulate. While teaching qualitative research online is not a matter of simply adjusting the syllabus to the online platform, it is possible to incorporate activities that can help students learn the skills and knowledge and develop the habits that we might want qualitative researchers to develop. Group work and problem-based learning strategies are particularly useful for online platforms. It reduces the isolation that students might face and links them to online communities of practice. Problem-based learning brings the issues and challenges of fieldwork to the forefront and students can, in groups, solve real problems that arise in their field experiences. Problem-based learning approaches often appeal to learners who enjoy puzzles, detective work, and moving fluidly from a micro to a macro and back to a micro level.

Helping students understand the concept of ambiguity, and learn to adjust to the types of ambiguity researchers face, can often be a pedagogical challenge. Faculty might benefit from making use of what we know about group dynamics and team building to help guide some pedagogical decisions. For example, are there activities or assignments that incorporate the forming, storming, norming, performing, and adjourning stages of group development (Tuckman & Jensen, 1977) in a way that is advantageous to simultaneously learning various dimensions of the research process for novice researchers? Can we be more intentional with building collaborative learning spaces for novice researchers? Panitz and Panitz (1998) offer a productive way to distinguish between collaborative learning spaces and cooperative learning spaces whereby collaborative is more student centered and they have more agency for directing their collective learning. Some examples of using these approaches in the context of teaching qualitative inquiry would include using a workshop design and/or incorporating studio pedagogies. These approaches may also lend themselves to an increased emphasis on experiential learning that uses classroom time in a variety of innovative ways. We refer to these simply as "exercises" because they are designed to engage students in the classroom using simulations, active problem-based scenarios, reflective activities, and/or help produce approximations of being a researcher in the field.

At times, faculty move to the other end of the spectrum and instead design courses that lead with theory and in-depth reading and contemplation. Often, very little experiential learning is used with this approach but rather it emphasizes readings (journal articles, books, and dissertations) that provide exemplars from within the qualitative research literature. Students' main activity is to analyze the readings and to raise potential practical questions from the exemplars they are studying. This approach is often effective for developing critical reading and analysis skills.

General Course Design Principles

Considering the various approaches that can be used to teach qualitative research courses, we now move into considering how the course design literature may offer us further opportunities to fine-tune qualitative inquiry courses.

Knowing the Learner: Countering and Working with the Resistant Learner

Knowing who the learner is or who the students are in a classroom is fundamental to teaching. Students can resist learning qualitative research for a number of reasons. For example, research methods courses are often cited by students as being boring, scary, or uncomfortable (Gray, 2013). As a way to counter such negative attitudes toward research, some scholars suggest pedagogical strategies that use materials drawn from popular culture to appeal to students as "pedagogic hooks," a process that is "fundamental work, central to bringing learners into the activity of researchers so that they might see or know research in engaging ways" (Lewthwaite & Nind, 2016, p. 421). Graham and Schuwerk (2017) suggest using episodes of *Undercover Boss* as a way to introduce or reinforce characteristics of qualitative research. Students could first learn or read or listen to a lecture on characteristics of qualitative research and then view, in groups, an episode of *Undercover Boss* (available on YouTube) and find those characteristics. Graham and Schuwerk found this strategy to be effective with assuaging student fears of research and allowed them to understand and apply what it means to do research in different contexts.

Inviting Students into a Community of Learning

Howard and Brady (2015) describe a constructivist pedagogical approach to teaching social science methods that focused on four strands. The first was to know the learners and where they stood in terms of their fears and understanding of research methods, similar to most pedagogical approaches. The second strand or pedagogical principle that they emphasized was to portray research methods as a contested field. The third was to provide space for students to choose a methodological approach that aligned with their personal beliefs regarding knowledge, and the fourth was to encourage students to think in terms of research as conversations or ongoing dialogues. The second and fourth principles mentioned here provide an entry for students to engage with debates that can lead to exploring the different ways in which scholars have approached the same issues or problems in the qualitative research process. In addition, engaging in conversations with peers can lead to awareness of their participation as part of a community of learners. As faculty teaching qualitative research, similarly, we are engaged in both the act of teaching as well as in pedagogical learning.

Reflection or Reflective Practices

Faculty new to teaching qualitative research courses will find they need to make decisions about the course structure, material, assessment, and topics that they intend to teach. The scholarship of teaching and learning has emphasized *reflection* as a key centerpiece of good teaching that can be used to explore the thinking of the teacher with that of the topic, the students, and the method used to facilitate the learning (Kreber, Castleden, Erfani, & Wright, 2005; McKeachie, 2013; Schon, 1987). The questions below, adapted from our own teaching, can serve as prompts for a reflective or ideas journal that can help one keep track of the different ideas that might be encountered. When we are asked to teach a new course, we typically like to write down some ideas or create an ideas list of things that we need to do to prepare. We share some of those questions below and hope they will be adapted to each individual taste and requirement. We suggest that faculty keep a teaching journal in which they can write notes to draw from and reflect on their pedagogy. Other suggestions may be to try audio- or videotaping a lesson to examine one's own teaching in detail and to engage others teaching similar courses to view and provide feedback to one another.

Exercise 2.1 may help structure some of the prethinking a faculty member could use when designing a course.

Faculty Reflective Journal Exercise 2.1. Prior to Teaching the Course

GOAL: Reflections on what I know and what I need to know.

Choose a journal that appeals to you—one that you will regard as a friend—as you write about your own thoughts and creative ideas, and keep track of your own learning.

The following exercise will take you about an hour. You need not do the entire exercise at one time. Usually these questions form the backbone of a course. Questions to write about:

1. Who is my audience?
   The course will be structured differently depending on whether the audience is undergraduate or graduate, this is a course in a sequence of courses, or is the only stand-alone course offered.

2. Do I have access to course outlines and syllabi in qualitative research that I might examine?

Having access to what previous instructors have taught can be instructive and useful as a starting point and at times can help one make decisions, even if they are about what one does not want to do.

3. What main topics do I want this course to cover?

A list of main topics can be long at first and edited later as the syllabus comes together.

4. What activities do I want to include or exclude?

This depends on the types of field research activities you might want to structure for students and your reasons for doing so. The suggestions in this book can offer a useful starting point.

A related issue to consider is whether you want students to analyze the data they gathered for a small-scale project or provide appropriate data for them to analyze. Both approaches have advantages and disadvantages. Students might be more engaged in analyzing their own datasets—however, the data might be inadequate for deep analysis. Data provided by faculty from their own research might be richer and allow for in-depth analyses and yet might be less engaging for students since it is not their own project. However, for reiterative practice purposes, providing data may be necessary since student data are likely to be gathered on a small scale.

5. What is my pedagogical approach?

Do I want to lecture, structure my classroom as discussion-oriented spaces that are also democratic, or activity based, or a little of everything? What balance do I want to maintain among different ways in which content is presented, explored, and discovered?

6. What are my assessment criteria?

How will I know whether students have learned what I intended them to learn in the course? This question will lead you to think about what assignments you want to create and how you want to assess them.

Brainstorm assignments for the course and brainstorm pedagogical strategies appropriate to teaching the particular concept, topic, and audience.

7. How much time will I need to plan my course and the sequence?

A standard time suggested by several scholars for preparing for a new course varies from 3 months to 4 weeks.

8. Do I have a large class with a teaching assistant?

If this is the case, then it may involve working with and training the graduate assistant or teaching assistants to grade field notes, lead discussion groups, establish criteria for independent and consultative decision making, and so on. Of course, each institution may have particular policies that guide what is considered appropriate work for a graduate or teaching assistant, and faculty ought to seek out the guidance of department chairs or others who can help interpret the policies. This will ensure that the Family Educational Rights and Privacy Act (FERPA) and other student protections are not jeopardized.

Exercise 2.2 provides another collection of prompts for self-assessment that can lead to next steps in the course design process.

Faculty Reflective Journal Exercise 2.2. Planning to Teach

GOAL: To start thinking about teaching qualitative research and prepare to teach.

Further questions to think about that are related to faculty development include:

1. What is my comfort level with teaching this course and how can I gain more confidence?
2. What can I learn while teaching this course?
3. How can I model learning while teaching this course?
4. Can I consider and plan a research project that I carry out while students are doing their projects as a way to demonstrate shared learning goals with the students?

Exercise 2.3 is representative of the types of ongoing weekly reflections that prove helpful during the semester in which the course is being taught.

Faculty Reflective Journal Exercise 2.3. Thinking about Teaching

GOAL: Weekly reflection on pedagogy.

WEEKLY JOURNAL ENTRY

A journal entry every week after teaching the class can enhance faculty development. Below, we offer different prompts for weekly journal entries with the caveat to break free from these prompts and just write freely if that works best for you.

Journal Writing Prompts

- First day of class—what I learned about the students. (Week 1 of the course)
- One challenge I faced this week in my teaching. (Week 2)
- One teaching moment. (Week 3)
- A journal article or reading that particularly resonated with students or that they particularly disliked. (Week 4)

- A new article that I read that taught me something about research methods or teaching. (Week 5)
- What is going well in my class? (Week 6)
- What can go better in my class? (Week 7)
- What can I do to give feedback so that students use it as a learning tool? (Week 8)
- What can I do differently?/What new pedagogical styles can I model? (Week 9)
- Something new I read that I can use in class. (Week 10)
- How can I assess student progress? (Week 11)
- What are some unique features of teaching qualitative research? (Week 12)
- What have I learned so far in my teaching? (Week 13)
- What has gone well this semester?/What will I do differently next time? (Week 14)

Assessment and evaluation or feedback and grading are important areas to contemplate while designing a course, yet in most cases faculty report needing experience with teaching a course one or two times before they are able to settle into a system that is manageable for their time constraints and productive for the students. It often takes high experimentation before you are able to find the right proportion. We all grapple with the realities of competing demands on our time and available energy for these labor-intensive tasks. Highly individualized feedback would pedagogically be best, yet literally impossible in most circumstances. There are, however, building blocks you can put in place to help increase the overall effectiveness of the assessment and evaluation plan you design. We offer 10 suggestions for how assessment and evaluation can be approached.

1. Strive for alignment among course goals, objectives, assignments, and assessment and evaluation. This ought to be accompanied by a philosophy of grading that is shareable with the students. For example, how would you answer these binary questions in relation to your course design? And how does your answer show up in your course design?

Is it possible for all students in my class to succeed or only a select few? Do I diversify my teaching methods or rely on one dominant method? Do I reward team problem solving among students or will I reward independent work?

The work you do to improve alignment will help increase student readiness for the types of formative and summative feedback you provide throughout the course

2. Be sensitive to the rhythms of the semester calendar. What weeks can you push harder and what weeks need a little less? How do you help students get ready for and anticipate the amount of time and energy particular kinds of in-class tasks and/or out-of-class assignments might require? Can you help them forecast in an effort to impact their individual planning?

3. Create assignments that are incremental, linked, and move the students toward the culminating final project. Make this process transparent for students so they can build a mental map for how the week-to-week work is assisting them with the final project. Can you create a visual chart or diagram that represents these linkages in a way that will show the skills and dispositions your course objectives have announced are essential components of the course? Can the students easily trace back to which course objectives are being worked on for each incremental assignment?

4. Develop rubrics to be shared with students to help guide their learning and specifically what skills and dispositions they ought to be focusing on for each assignment. Rubrics help to make clear levels of success for each complex task or process associated with each assignment.

5. Make effective use of oral and written peer-review processes. Peer review for students encompasses an array of essential learnings, including sharpening their analytical, communication, and writing skills. It can often help to provide some "training" to students about how to conduct a peer review in general and then specifically for the types of work to be reviewed in your course.

6. Task and time management strategies for "grading" are by far the most complained about aspect of teaching qualitative inquiry courses. Pragmatically blocking out the time needed in your weekly schedule to read and provide feedback is an involved and complex process. Depending on how many students, what type of assignments, how you have structured the rubric, what type(s) of feedback will be required to keep students progressing forward, and in what form(s) will the feedback arrive (e.g., hand written, electronically written, sketch notes for a more visual effect, audio notes, face-to-face meetings in your office or using Skype, FaceTime, or Zoom) are all items to take into consideration to help estimate the amount of time needed for grading. In addition, you may incorporate into the delivery of graded assignments "next steps" or encouragement for continuing to improve upon the skills and dispositions desired in relation to the course objectives. All of this must be

carved out in relation to the various other demands on your time and is often further conditioned by your location in the tenure and promotion cycle.

7. Consider the pros and cons of providing exemplary models or examples ahead of assignments from prior students who have taken the course (with permission) and/or the published literature. This may be appropriate or useful in some cases but not all.

8. Consider whether you will implement a revise and resubmit option for some or all assignments. What are the advantages or disadvantages?

9. Consider whether your grading system will be numerical/points based, letter-grade based, narrative/comments based, or come combination of these means to communicate the level or degree of obtaining the course objectives. Consider this question for both the formative assessments and the summative evaluation (overall grade for the course).

10. Seek out colleagues who are teaching the same or similar courses to construct a peer group that can offer advice, critique, and support as you consider the impact of various assessment and evaluation systems for your course. Seek faculty who are willing to share syllabi and the stories that accompany their syllabi—the backstory of creation, the go-live story as it unfolded, and the poststory as they unpack the overall effectiveness of the course design on their students.

A note about online teaching: The challenges of teaching research methods online cannot be minimized. Yet, it is possible to re-create the large-group back-and-forth dialogue in online groups. Our experiences in using videos, Skype, and Zoom, and allowing students to use these to interact with one another, greatly enhanced the discussions in some groups, while in other groups, students chose to remain in asynchronous mode and had rich, detailed discussions in that format—the flexibility it affords students is a positive. In terms of giving feedback and contributing to the discussions, faculty may find it easier to give feedback to groups rather than individuals. Other tips for online teaching include:

1. Time management awareness for faculty and students. Create a schedule for reading and responding online so that feedback is timely, even if brief. This can help students feel connected to the faculty in an online course. Similarly, a suggested note to students about how to manage time with reading and writing within the week or module has been well received by students.

2. Give short but effective feedback regularly using varying formats—audio, video, or text. Setting up a system by which students know when to expect feedback also helps students feel connected to instructors in online courses. This will also help faculty to schedule their time for giving feedback.

3. Experiment with participation in discussion forums to create the right presence that will encourage and not stifle conversation among students. Asking questions, rewording questions to move the discussions in different directions, providing resources or evidence, and summarizing discussions briefly are all roles that faculty can adopt. Be sure to participate, even if such roles are delegated to students.

4. Create lessons in multiple formats. You might want to ensure that any introduction or lecture notes are in text as well as in video or audio format to accommodate students' learning styles. While this might seem daunting, a lecture or note can simply be read out.

5. Make any PowerPoint presentations or notes interactive. Create a brief worksheet for viewing PowerPoints and intersperse the presentation with questions that students have to answer on the worksheet as they proceed with their viewing.

These examples of the main elements of different types of syllabi are ideas of how one can approach course design and think through the purpose and rationale for the pedagogical approach outlined.

CHAPTER SUMMARY ● ● ● ● ● ● ● ● ● ● ● ●

Overall, this chapter examined the various approaches to teaching qualitative inquiry, offered ways to use course design principles to guide the building of courses, and provided guiding concepts for how to start the process of teaching. The next chapter reexamines approaches to teaching qualitative inquiry from the perspective of holistic pedagogy.

Sample Syllabi Templates (Face-to-Face, Workshop and Studio Based, Online)

EXAMPLE 1. This example provides some elements included in a syllabus for a face-to-face, theory-driven approach to an introduction to qualitative inquiry.

COURSE TITLE: THEORETICAL FOUNDATIONS OF QUALITATIVE RESEARCH—AN INTRODUCTION

Course Description

This course is designed to build students' foundational knowledge of qualitative theories and methodologies and demonstrate the complex nature of doing this type of work. Students are expected to read and critique various theories, frameworks, ideologies, and methods of qualitative research. Students will learn about the epistemological and paradigmatic foundations of qualitative research, and how to differentiate and understand the interconnections between them. We engage in a study of qualitative methodologies through our class discussions and activities, personal and professional experiences, and graded assignments.

Course Goals

- Gain a clear understanding of qualitative theories and research methods.
- Identify and explain ideologies that contribute to the complex nature of qualitative research. Grapple with the construction, implementation, and evaluation of particular research methods. Identify and create qualitative research questions based on contemporary educational or social problems.
- Clarify individual goals and choices regarding students' research projects.

Course Objectives

The students will:

- Review, critique, and identify theories of qualitative research in examples of qualitative reports or articles.
- Become critical readers of qualitative research with regard to the researcher's chosen methodologies.

Assignments

1. Submit weekly reaction papers to the readings in the course.
2. Submit one example every 3 weeks of an article of your choice written from a particular paradigm. Explain what the paradigm is and what you learned about the theory of qualitative research utilized in the article.
3. Final paper. Write a paper where you create three imaginary studies of a

particular topic of interest to you. Use any three paradigms (e.g., postpositivist, critical, feminist, interpretive, postmodern) and include information in each of the studies about the purpose of the study, design, data analysis, and the relationship of researcher to participants. Write a summary of how your study changed with the change in paradigms.

Suggested Texts

Denzin, N., & Lincoln, Y. S. (2012). *The landscape of qualitative research*. Thousand Oaks, CA: SAGE.

Eisner, E. (1998). *The enlightened eye: Qualitative inquiry and the enhancement of educational practice*. Upper Saddle River, NJ: Merrill Press.

Swaminathan, R., & Mulvihill, T. M. (2017). *Critical approaches to questions in qualitative research*. London: Routledge.

Willis, J. (2007). *Foundations of qualitative research: Interpretive and critical approaches*. Thousand Oaks, CA: SAGE.

Recommended Readings

Creswell, J. W. (2013). *Qualitative inquiry and research design: Choosing among five approaches*. (3rd ed.). Thousand Oaks, CA: SAGE.

Glesne, C. E. (2006). *Becoming qualitative researchers*. New York: Pearson.

Schwandt, T. (2001). *Dictionary of qualitative inquiry* (2nd ed.). Thousand Oaks, CA: SAGE.

Stake, R. E. (1995). *The art of case study research*. Thousand Oaks, CA: SAGE.

· ·

EXAMPLE 2. This example provides some elements included in a syllabus using workshop and studio pedagogies for a face-to-face graduate seminar on ethnography and education.

EDST 660 SEC. 001 FALL 2017: SEMINAR—ETHNOGRAPHY AND EDUCATION

Thalia M. Mulvihill, PhD, Professor of Social Foundations and Higher Education

Course Description

The purpose of this course is to conduct an investigation into current qualitative research paradigms, models, and methods of inquiry related to ethnography. We pursue this investigation by engaging in advanced qualitative inquiry (skill-building) workshops, institutional review board (IRB)-approved ethnographic fieldwork, and through rigorous seminar discussions. This course employs immersive, studio, and hybrid pedagogies that emphasize learning by doing and requires a well-thought-out qualitative inquiry project at the start of the course.

Course Objectives

1. To provide students an opportunity to identify and describe current issues in conducting qualitative research.
2. To assist students in developing a general knowledge of qualitative research paradigms, methods, and modes of inquiry related to ethnography as they are used by educators and social scientists.
3. To provide students with an opportunity to engage in IRB-approved field-work.
4. To provide students with an opportunity to develop data collection, data analysis, and research report-writing skills.
5. To encourage students to develop strong and vital collegial relationships with their peers.

Assignments

1. **Readings**

   The readings used in this course come from a variety of sources.

   Required

   Bogdan, R. C., & Biklen, S. K. (2007). *Qualitative research for education: An introduction to theory and methods* (5th ed.). Boston: Allyn & Bacon.

   Creswell, J. W. (2013). *Qualitative inquiry and research design: Choosing among five approaches.* (3rd ed.). Thousand Oaks, CA: SAGE.

   Leavy, P. (2014). *The Oxford handbook of qualitative research.* New York: Oxford University Press.

   Course documents: Other readings distributed by the professor electronically on Blackboard.

   Recommended

   Denzin, N. K., & Lincoln, Y. S. (2011). *The SAGE handbook of qualitative research: Educational anthropology and research methodolgy* (4th ed.). Thousand Oaks, CA: SAGE.

   Holman Jones, S., Adams, T. E., & Ellis, C. (Eds.). (2013). *Handbook of autoethnography.* New York: Routledge.

   Mulvihill, T. M., & Swaminathan, R. (2017). *Critical approaches to life writing methods in qualitative research.* New York: Routledge.

   Savin-Baden, M., & Howell Major, C. (2013). *Qualitative research: The essential guide to theory and practice.* New York: Routledge.

   Swaminathan, R., & Mulvihill, T. M. (2017). *Critical approaches to questions in qualitative research.* London: Routledge.

   Wolcott, H. F. (2009). *Writing up qualitative research* (3rd ed.). Thousand Oaks, CA: SAGE.

2. **Writing Assignments**

   a. **Reaction Papers** (see course agenda for due dates—five total; 10%)

      This writing assignment is designed to keep you actively writing about your ideas in relation to the readings. Reaction papers should be 500–800 words in length and deal with the issues raised in the readings due for that day. This word limitation is designed to help you refine your thinking. I will respond with written comments and return these papers to you using the following rating scale: outstanding = 2 points, good = 1 point, needs improvement or no submission = 0 points.

   b. **Electronic Discussions** (one per week; 15%)

      You are expected to contribute regularly to electronic discussions posted on Blackboard. The discussions are, for example, continuations of in-class discussions and provide further opportunities to explore course readings and course themes. Contributions are expected to be in the form of original posts and responses to the posts of your colleagues in the course. You are required to make one original post (at least 500 words) and respond to at least two posts (response posts) contributed by your colleagues (at least 300 words each). (A total of three posts per discussion.)

      These electronic discussions are opportunities for you to:

      - Demonstrate your ability to analyze course material.
      - Demonstrate your ability to construct meaningful questions.
      - Demonstrate your ability to construct a collaborative learning environment.
      - Demonstrate your ability to share your learning with colleagues in the course.

   c. **Researcher's Journal** (one per week; 15%)

      You will make weekly entries related to your fieldwork in an electronic journal posted on Blackboard.

   d. **Final Project** (60%)

      You will prepare a final research report related to your fieldwork.

· ·

EXAMPLE 3. This example provides some elements included in a syllabus for an online introduction to a qualitative inquiry course.

INTRODUCTION TO QUALITATIVE RESEARCH (ONLINE COURSE)

Course Description

The purpose of the course is to provide an understanding of qualitative research methods in the cultural foundations of education that allows you to write a master's thesis or a research paper. To this end, we discuss different methods for conducting research, what drives the research methodology, and what types of questions constitute research questions. This course addresses both theoretical and practical dimensions of conducting research. While many research methods exist, and we touch upon some of them, this course primarily focuses on different types of qualitative research. The course addresses issues such as the ethics and politics of research as well as specific and practical considerations of research activities. The course also provides an opportunity to think critically about research, share your thoughts, learn things from your fellow classmates, and conduct a simulated qualitative research project. The course is designed with flexibility so that you can develop projects that suit your own academic needs. The workload in the course is somewhat extensive—however, I hope that you find the course intrinsically interesting and valuable.

Course Objectives

By the end of the course it is expected that you will be able to:

- Explain the difference between qualitative, quantitative, and mixed-methods research designs and identify how they complement one another and when one might be more appropriate than the other.
- Articulate the benefits and limitations of each approach.
- Reflect on ethical issues related to research.
- Conduct a literature review on a topic of interest.
- Be able to read and critically evaluate qualitative research studies and determine their strengths and weaknesses.
- Develop a qualitative research project related to your interests.
- Write a research report based on a literature review and field research.

Course Guidelines

1. As this class is fully online, it is dependent on everyone's commitment to participating fully and thoughtfully in discussion and in sharing with one another what you are learning from your own projects. As a general rule, always treat people the same way as you would like to be treated.

2. In completing your coursework, always challenge yourself to learn new things and grow as a person. Challenge yourself and your classmates to think of things in ways you/they never have before.

3. In an online course, you are what you write. As this is an academic course, it is important to complete assignments using correct grammar, spelling, and netiquette. Texting language used in course assignments will not be accepted. *Appropriate language in e-mail correspondence is also expected. When e-mailing me please be sure to use punctuation, capital letters, spelling, grammar, and netiquette.*

Instructional Materials

Required

Creswell, J. W. (2013). *Qualitative inquiry and research design: Choosing among five approaches* (3rd ed.). Thousand Oaks, CA: SAGE.

Mulvihill, T. M., & Swaminathan, R. (2017). *Critical approaches to life writing methods in qualitative research.* New York: Routledge.

Swaminathan, R., & Mulvihill, T. M. (2017). *Critical approaches to questions in qualitative research.* New York: Routledge.

Additional materials, like lecture notes, voiceover PowerPoint presentations, required articles, and supplementary video clips, will be posted on our course site's content page in D2L. *Content will, in most cases, be available several weeks in advance.*

Course Expectations

During this semester, in this online class, we will utilize mainly asynchronous learning. I will be available via Skype for meetings and for Skype chat, and will set up chat in D2L or Google Hangouts for us to meet when possible.

- Students are expected to read the assigned readings and actively participate in discussions each week, and other activities as assigned. This means logging in at least three times per week. Expect to spend between 9 and 12 hours per week for this course.
- Students are expected to post assignments on the date due.

Structure of the Course

Every week, the course comprises both analyzing the readings and learning the "how to's" of conducting research. In addition, we will learn about issues like the politics of research, gender and race issues in research, action research, and the politics and ethics of fieldwork. We will also share field experiences and discuss them in relation to the issues raised in the readings. Some guest presentations may also take place.

With regard to the readings and discussion board: Although the discussions cannot completely ignore the substantive content of the article we discuss, the emphasis of the talk should be on the theoretical orientation, organization, form, and style of the manuscript. Some questions that might be addressed include:

What was the author trying to accomplish?

How did he or she proceed?

Is it a successful article? Why?

For whom was it written?

How does the article fit with the time in which it was written?

What are its weaknesses?

Is it convincing? Well written?

What theoretical perspective was employed?

How were the data displayed?

How would you evaluate the article?

Would you give it a high rating? Why?

Most of the discussion board participation asks you to apply what you have read.

Assignments

1. *Discussion board participation.* This course requires thoughtful preparation on your part. Your attentive reading to the texts and your participation in class will earn you points. You may also be asked to comment critically on readings, analyze each other's writing, or comment on class discussions or activities. With regard to discussion board participation, you will be given specific tasks to accomplish every week/module. These can include video analysis, text analysis, critical reading, and blogging on a class site designed for this purpose.

2. *Every Sunday the discussion board for the following week will be open. The discussion boards will close every Saturday at midnight.* Some course modules will continue for a 2-week period to allow you time to get your reading and writing completed. In all such cases, I will provide you with deadlines and guidelines. Be sure to adhere to them so that we can have productive online class exchanges.

At least one of your posts needs to be completed by Wednesday at midnight and the remainder by Friday at midnight. Every week or module, you will receive some guidance on how to manage your time for reading, writing, conducting your simulated field research, and participating in this course.

3. *Online discussions.* The course is divided into topic-centered units. You are expected to complete reading assignments and participate actively in online discussions. During the asynchronous online discussions, you are required to respond to questions posted by classmates, and to review and comment on the responses of others. A quality message is two to three paragraphs in length that includes ideas from the readings and/or personal experience. Quality messages can be in response to the posted questions (instructor or student created) or replies posted by others (instructor or students). You are required to post specific numbers of messages per discussion period. Every week, except for the first, you are required to post at least twice—once by Wednesday at midnight and the second by Friday at midnight. There will be several activities for you to complete during the semester.

A total of 10 points per week (except in certain cases where the number of points will be indicated) are possible. I will grade the discussions based on the following rubric:

8–10 Points

The student posted the required amount of messages (or more) and interacted with his or her group members.

The student made timely and appropriate comments that were reflective
and critical in nature.

The student made reference to the course content and/or personal experiences related to the topic matter.

Detail and language demonstrate an understanding of the major ideas
and concepts.
Questions indicate a high level of analysis and insight.
Analysis indicates critical thinking and thoughtful reflections.
The student made few or no grammar or spelling errors.

5–7 Points

The student posted the required amount of messages and interacted with
his or her group members.

The student made appropriate comments, but they lacked depth.

The student made reference to the course content and/or personal experience related to the topic matter.

The student may have made some grammar and spelling errors.

1–4 Points

The student may not have posted the required amount of messages or did
not interact with his or her group members.

The student may not have added anything new to the conversation.

The student may not have referenced the course content or referenced it in
a faulty manner.

The student may have committed spelling and grammar errors that make
his or her messages hard to read.

0 Points

The student has not posted any messages.

4. *Research project.* This is the main project for this course and will be a
simulated study because a real-life project would require you to gather far more
data than the time frame for this course allows. You will be required to post
selections of your data and analysis to the discussion board for peer comments
and reflection. The project leads up to a final paper/report that you will submit
on the last day of class.

CHAPTER 3

It's Never Too Early to Start "Thinking Qualitatively"

Since students new to qualitative research methods courses come in with preconceived ideas of research, it is important for teachers of qualitative research to engage them in reflection and awareness exercises. Engaging students helps them to understand their values and belief systems and the potential impact of the same on their approaches to research.

In this chapter, we:

- Address the ways in which teachers of qualitative research can facilitate student awareness of their own taken-for-granted assumptions of research.

- Describe holistic pedagogy and advance an argument for why this approach is essential to the nature of teaching qualitative inquiry.

- Discuss how faculty, by adopting a holistic pedagogical approach, can help students "think qualitatively" and, in a practical sense, identify a research question that can be approached qualitatively.

Using a Holistic Approach to Thinking Pedagogically about Teaching Qualitative Research

To be awake is to take risks, to see things that you probably would not want to see. We have to teach that—an awareness, a courage to see. Without it, we'll just be for profit, and not for meaning.
—MAXINE GREENE, 1978, quoted in Gentry (2011)

Greene (1978) emphasized the need for "wide-awakeness" in order to counter the pervasive indifference and apathy of our time. She suggests that the way to overcome such feelings of apathy or indifference is "through conscious endeavor on the part of individuals to keep themselves awake, to think about their condition in the world, to inquire into the forces that appear to dominate them, to interpret the experiences they are having day by day" (p. 44). We apply these concepts to teaching and learning qualitative research where an attention to awareness through inquiry is essential for the student and educator alike. Palmer (2010) says that the right questions to ask about one's teaching are the "who" questions, and not so much the "how to teach" or the "what to teach" questions. "Who" is the self that teaches and how does that quality of selfhood inform the way we relate to students, colleagues, and the world? To keep these questions central to the pedagogical endeavor, we advocate and practice a holistic pedagogical approach that focuses on the inner landscape of the teaching self and includes intellect, the spirit, and the emotions of the teacher (Miller, 2000, 2005; Nakagawa, 2000). hooks (1994) shares her most personal insights into the dynamics of teaching in a college classroom and narrates her educational transgressions for all educators to contemplate their purpose and the means they use to achieve their pedagogical goals. Bhattacharya (*http://kakali. org*) offers an abundance of rich material around contemplative practice, mindfulness, and qualitative inquiry (Bhattacharya, 2017), and has tapped into the possibilities qualitative researchers have to powerfully confront colonialist and hegemonic thinking (Bhattacharya, 2016). This is just a sampling of those who have written about pedagogical approaches that have direct relevance for the types of thinking faculty can engage in as they contemplate their own identity as teachers and the work involved in preparing researchers. Preparing the next generation of qualitative researchers requires that those of us who teach these courses continue to challenge and confront our own assumptions and to invite our students into the dialogue about the continuous nature of this type of reflexivity for all researchers. In this book, we are advocating for a holistic pedagogical approach.

What Is a Holistic Pedagogy? And Why Is It Needed?

A holistic approach is an integrated approach that encompasses the whole—the mind, body, and inner spirit of the learner and teacher (Miller, 2005). A holistic pedagogy is in line with recent work in the study of teaching and learning where scholars address the importance of examining multiple dimensions of teacher and learner identities (Korthagen, 2004). This involves learning about the environment within which one teaches, knowing the learners, responding to situations, and creating possibilities for critical thinking and growth (Korthagen, 2004; Patel, 2003). A holistic approach involves teaching in ways that acknowledge multiple modes of acquiring knowledge—for example, learning with the body, learning through reason, and learning through contemplation. Qualitative research involves the acquisition and interpretation of knowledge from all these dimensions and a holistic approach to qualitative pedagogy frames teaching qualitative research as a complex and creative endeavor. In teaching qualitative research, we find this approach most appropriate since it validates, challenges, and addresses the myriad facets of students' experiences in the act of research. It calls for layered nuances of awareness and reflection for the educator and the student alike. It challenges students to be attentive to nuances of power, to be aware of the purposes of research in the public interest (Ladson-Billings & Tate, 2006), and to be awake to the possibilities of surprise and creativity in the research act. In addition, a holistic approach moves away from a relationship of hierarchical domination to one of actualization (Eisler, 2005). A hierarchy of actualization recognizes that a classroom is rarely horizontal, but that a partnership of learning and reciprocity is possible between the educator and the student. Through a holistic pedagogical approach, educators can facilitate learners to be reflective and reflexive as they see themselves in the act of learning, discovery, and questioning for knowledge generation and personal and professional growth. The basis of holistic pedagogy is that teaching is a social activity involving interactions both between and among the students and educator. A holistic educator is also assumed to be a learner, and the interaction between the student and the educator impacts not only the student but the teacher as well. In the practice of holistic education, the educator would want to facilitate the development of the learner into an independent, confident, critical thinker while continuously reflecting on the act of teaching. In the next section, we outline some key characteristics of holistic pedagogy that can inform educators teaching qualitative research.

Key Characteristics of Holistic Pedagogy for Teaching Qualitative Research

We have distilled **seven** characteristics of holistic pedagogy that apply to the teaching of qualitative research: (1) inclusivity and transdisciplinarity; (2) concern with social justice; (3) inquiry based; (4) open and flexible curriculum and approach; (5) concern with knowing or investigating the self; (6) reciprocal learning based on a relationship of care; and (7) use of dialogue and silence, solitude, and community.

Below we describe each of these characteristics in some detail, and provide starter examples:

1. *Holistic pedagogy involves an approach to curriculum that is inclusive and transdisciplinary.* Applying these characteristics to the teaching of qualitative research means drawing attention to the transdisciplinary nature of qualitative research. Books from different disciplines—namely, nursing, sociology, political science, social work, and education—can add to students' experiences of what qualitative research looks like from different perspectives. By including examples of studies from different disciplines, educators can fuel the research imagination and provide opportunities for students to think laterally.

2. *Holistic pedagogy is also concerned with social justice.* Teaching qualitative research, particularly from a critical framework, means centralizing social justice as a key reason for conducting research. This includes guiding students to pay attention to issues of power, hierarchy, race, and culture throughout the research process. As a pedagogical approach, it utilizes the classroom as a democratic space where the hierarchy of power relations between the educator and the students is discussed and mitigated to the extent possible. Such a pedagogy also demands that the educator be attentive to the nuances of power relations among students so that the principles of inclusivity are practiced as part of the intent toward social justice. Working from this pedagogical stance helps the students stay mindful and attentive to the forms of power that are present and how they operate in the social world. Incorporating these discussions into the qualitative research methods class helps students sharpen their observation skills and improves their abilities to ask meaningful research questions.

3. *Holistic pedagogy centralizes inquiry-based thinking.* In teaching qualitative research, an inquiring, curious mind that continually asks questions is essential. Questioning also implies skepticism along with curiosity so that the learner and the educator strive to take nothing for granted. Instead, they seek evidence as they formulate ideas and connections between phenomena. In the application of teaching, this means the holistic educator creates opportunities through situations and scenarios for students in the classroom that encourage questioning. This could involve role-playing, debates, panel discussions, Socratic dialogues, and cases that can be used to structure critical thinking and questioning.

4. *Holistic pedagogy has an open and flexible curriculum and approach.* In teaching qualitative research, this means structuring the curriculum to the needs of the students. One way of remaining learner

centered is to offer a range of reading choices. Another is to structure the curriculum so that there are opportunities for students to collaborate as well as work alone. A third way is to respond to learners' needs and be sensitive to where students are in their own development and understanding of qualitative research. This aspect of holistic pedagogy requires the educator to encounter all student questions, resistances, and reactions to the learning process with an open posture. In other words, the educator must readily interpret all student behavior and actions as points of discovery that will help direct the next series of successive actions the educator will take as the course evolves.

5. *Holistic pedagogy is concerned with knowing or investigating the self.* In teaching qualitative research, knowing the self is an ongoing inquiry and is usually referred to as the reflexive process. Applied to teaching, the educator uses reflexivity to question power relations in the classroom while finding ways to create spaces for all students to engage in dialogue across race and cultural lines. By examining the self, the educator encourages students to find commonality in difference and seek difference in commonality. The educator seeks to remain in the state that Freire (2000) referred to as "unfinished"—a state in which one is constantly seeking to grow and learn.

6. *Holistic education is concerned with reciprocal learning based on a relationship of care.* Qualitative pedagogy involves reciprocity and draws on Vygotsky's (1978) and other scholars' (Rosenshine & Meister, 1994; Williams, 2010) explanations of reciprocal teaching. Reciprocal teaching is a collaboration between educators and students where each learns from the other. In qualitative research, the classroom presents an opportunity for educators to reflect on teaching while also presenting opportunities to respond to students' diverse needs based on an ethic of care.

7. *Holistic education uses dialogue, silence, solitude, and community.* Pedagogies that are equally centered on silence and solitude as much as dialogue and community take into consideration the unconscious processes of the brain and the time to ponder so that new connections emerge after a period of contemplative inquiry. The contemplation we refer to here is the mindful yet energetic attention to new possibilities in qualitative research that can then be reflected in our teaching. These are distinct yet related experiences that can be woven together within the context of a course on qualitative inquiry.

The basic premise of holistic pedagogy is that teaching is a social activity involving interactions both between and among the students as well as the educator. A holistic educator is also assumed to be a learner and the interaction between the student and the educator impacts not only the student but the teacher as well. Often, teaching qualitative research involves working against novice researchers' starting assumptions wrapped in positivist thinking and ideas of what constitutes research. Often, students automatically assume that research is quantitative research that begins with a hypothesis and is relatively researcher-proof. And in much the same way, they consider empirical research to mean dealing with numbers only. Initial brainstorming sessions on topics of interest often bring up questions that have to do with surveys or comparing two groups or trying to get at the effects of a particular intervention. To begin altering this type of mind-set requires a shift in students' habitual ways of thinking and knowing the world. Thinking qualitatively is central to learning qualitative research. In the next sections, we explain what qualitative researchers mean by the phrase *thinking qualitatively,* and suggest ways to introduce and engage students in qualitative thinking.

What Does It Mean to Think Qualitatively?

Every semester, when we teach the qualitative research course, we can almost pinpoint the exact moment when students "get it." *Getting it* may be an ambiguous and unscholarly term, but as educators teaching qualitative research methods courses, we can relate to these "Aha!" moments when students' eyes light up. While we know when students get it after the fact, the challenge is to try to figure out what we mean by getting it—how to recognize it and communicate it to our students. The "it" in "getting it" refers to what we have come to term *qualitative thinking.* To us, qualitative thinking is more than methods—it is a perspective, a way of seeing, and a way of wondering about the social world. Scholars have used the term *qualitative thinking* in different ways. According to Agar (2004), qualitative thinking is about a "way of looking at a problem, not just about academic theory and method and research design." Morse (1994), who first used the term *qualitative thinking,* and Agar (1999) both explained what qualitative thinking would look like by describing its features.

Agar (1999) pinpoints three characteristics of qualitative thinking, all of which emerge in the act of doing qualitative research. The first is the idea that questions occur during the act of doing research that one would not have thought of before entering the field. Researchers have to be prepared to be flexible and modify their research questions if they find that the field presents new ideas that are relevant and important for the overall purpose of the study. For example, in one research project, we wanted to find out about teachers' peer friendships only to discover that teachers do not define their working relationships as friendships. We needed to modify our question to get at the multiple roles and relations in which teachers see themselves. We also learned that the talk that teachers engaged in was found mostly in the teachers' lounge and therefore decided that participant observation along with interviews was the best way to examine teacher discourses in schools. Questions emerging in the field may therefore become the focal point of the research. In other words, researchers have to be prepared for new questions to arise in context.

The second characteristic is "abductive thinking." By that Agar (1999) refers to researchers' creative thinking when they try to explain what they observe in the field without resorting to preconceived ideas or concepts. Abductive thinking requires researchers to be open to making sense of what they see in the field by trying to make connections between events, incidents, or discussions. For example, one of us, in a project on collaboration in community settings, engaged in abductive thinking when we found that at community partnership meetings, the least vocal in the group were also the people with the most influence. A preconceived idea about leadership might have led us to think differently and assume that those participants who spoke most often were the leaders. However, in engaging in abductive thinking, we needed to pay attention to nuances that helped us to identify the group with the most influence or the quiet leaders.

The third characteristic is to examine data sources to build thematic story lines. Agar's (1999) definition leads the way in helping us understand what might constitute qualitative thinking. Saldana (2015) explains that qualitative thinking comprises a range of ways of thinking. These include Bloom's (1956) revised taxonomy of levels of thinking (Sousa, 2011)—namely, using creativity as well as symbolism, metaphors, and memory to lead researchers to a point where they coalesce their meaning making. Saldana (2015) refers to this process as "consolidation," or as a type of synthesis where snippets, brief actions, or focused conversations in the field all begin to merge together into a story that takes into account the different scenes. Richardson and St. Pierre (2005) clarify the activity referred to as "thinking qualitatively" as *inquiry,* a term that spurs us to act as inquirers. Inquiry is a continuous process, a "nomadic" process that takes researchers on a journey of discovery and encourages them to think deeply about what they encounter and make connections that they had not considered before. Qualitative thinking embraces a variety of ways of looking at the world as it occurs continuously throughout the research process. It includes a way of seeing, a sense of wonder, feelings of discomfort, and most crucial, a questioning attitude. To engage students and novice researchers in these types of qualitative thinking, educators can utilize experiential learning as well as dialogue and role play. Using multiple ways to teach can highlight and introduce students to different dimensions of qualitative research while giving them practice in thinking qualitatively.

Teaching Qualitative Thinking through Experiential Learning

Teaching qualitative thinking draws on creativity and the imagination as much as it draws on observation, perspective, and critical questioning. This means viewing the classroom, the students, and the teaching process itself from a "learning framework." Drawing on Dweck's (2006) work on *Mindset* and on Palmer's (2010) work with teachers, we are mindful of the continuous identity work and reflection we need to engage in as educators while teaching qualitative research. Building students' capacity for thinking qualitatively necessarily includes the affective domain, while we are mindful about the traps of disassociating thinking from emotions in the classroom. Qualitative thinking in this sense cannot be separated from qualitative fieldwork or from the analyses, and neither can thinking be disconnected from the emotions that might be stirred up during the processes.

Thinking qualitatively means learning how to experience and understand the social realities of others while simultaneously charting your own cognitive and emotional reactions to the lived experiences of others. Therefore, it is essential for novice researchers to have experiential components in their introduction to qualitative research. Whereas experiential learning has its roots in the scholarship of Dewey (1938) and Kolb and Kolb (2012), qualitative research has had a long history of experiential learning in the field. As teachers of qualitative research, we enter this liminal space with our students and help them validate the whole range of experiences and reactions they have and find ways to help them nurture more meaningful and nuanced understandings of others and self and the interactions between. Some entry points into these types of ongoing discussions might include "thought experiments" that are meant to help novice researchers become more discerning and more comfortable with the range of emotions they may encounter when engaged in "fieldwork."

Students new to research may be over- or underconcerned with how their participants might perceive them. They may become preoccupied with whether they are "liked" and find themselves drifting away from the necessary researcher's mantel; the role and related countenance that propels them forward to conduct the business of collecting data by developing a relational conversation or establishing the rapport needed in order to navigate a semistructured interview. Moments such as these are ripe for educators to use as places to reemphasize that thinking qualitatively means coming to terms with the initial discomforts of entering the field, establishing a trustworthy space where knowledge is co-constructed, and recognizing that thinking qualitatively demands a higher-order form of communication.

Engaging in even small-scale versions of pedagogical reflexivity—such as creating a set of field notes after each class session and then examining those data by conducting an analysis to break apart and then reconstitute the data, including the new and next-level questions you develop to help guide the shaping of the next class session—is an opportunity to model for students the benefits and difficulties of the reflexivity process. This type of intentional examination and reexamination of a sociocultural space (i.e., classroom) and a willingness to transparently share the self-examination process with the class can also be used as an opportunity to talk about discomfort and learning in the art of reflexivity while drawing attention to the parallel of being in the field for students. Learning to become reflexive requires novice researchers to encounter "the field" and to engage in the critical and creative thinking that is a hallmark of qualitative inquiry.

Field experiences (i.e., visits to the field that are not duration specific) or field exercises (i.e., shorter visits to the field meant to provide initial learning experiences for novice researchers where authentic questions are raised for further methodological examination) can stimulate thinking from different perspectives. These pedagogically focused field exercises are designed to help novice researchers build their capacity to see, question, wonder, and understand the field in the context of their own frames of reference and in a way that can be discussed in class, among peers/colleagues, to call forth further refinements of understanding of the relationship between self (researcher) and data from the social world (the field). Developing this type of conscious awareness is one of the foundations of qualitative thinking. This type of awareness requires students to learn to be attentive to nuances of power and relationships—to listen to what is not said and to examine what is absent or missing. Qualitative thinking requires framing the obvious and looking for traces of that which is less visible or vanishing. It involves becoming consciously aware of ways of thinking that we take for granted and to challenge areas rarely considered. This type of classroom exercise serves as practice sessions for eventual fieldwork and allows students to make mistakes, experiment, and discuss what they are learning in the company of their peers. The improvisational quality of these early experiences can help reinforce the iterative and emergent nature of this type of thinking and reinforce the necessity of peer conversations/debriefing.

In Exercises 3.1 and 3.2, we illustrate two practice exercises that can be used in the classroom to build novice researchers' skills of observation and reflexivity as they explore ways of "seeing" and "reflecting." After students complete these exercises, educators can hold debriefing sessions with students through reflection prompts and guided classroom discussions.

Classroom Exercise 3.1. Grocery Store

GOAL: To describe a familiar place as if it were new.

OUTCOMES: This activity helps students to understand how familiar spaces contain things they have often never noticed before. This draws their attention to activities going on in these spaces that they normally would not notice. By deliberately calling attention to those activities, it helps students to begin to see familiar spaces as if for the first time. It encourages curiosity, a key ingredient in research observation.

TIME: 20 minutes observation prior to class session and 20–30 minutes of in-class discussion.

GUIDELINES TO SHARE WITH STUDENTS: Go to a grocery store that you visit regularly. This time, as you buy a product of your choice, think about why you bought what you did, who are the people around you, and whether you feel comfortable here. Why or why not? What types of interactions take place at this store? What are some of the unwritten "rules" that are followed? For example, there could be a certain order of moving in aisles or waiting in line to buy bread. What are grocery store rules? Does everyone seem to know the rules? Think about what you could not do in a grocery store or what would be frowned upon. This will help you to understand in context some rules that govern behavior in grocery stores.

REFLECTION PROMPTS FOR STUDENTS: Share your thoughts about your visit to the grocery store with two peers in your class. Use the following prompts to jump-start a discussion:

1. What was different about this visit to a familiar grocery store?
2. What did you notice about the grocery store that you had previously not noticed?
3. What emotions did you notice in this familiar space both in yourself and around you?
4. What rules of grocery store shopping could you discern from your visit?
5. What role did your own prior experiences with grocery stores play in your sense making?

6. What assumptions did you hold about the people you expected to observe before entering the grocery store?

7. What assumptions do you think the people in the grocery store held about you when they saw you there?

8. Did you buy anything while you were there? Why or why not?

9. What questions about qualitative research and the role of the researcher emerged during your visit?

In Exercise 3.1, we shared an activity that allows students to begin to notice and observe new things in a familiar space, leading them to emotions of wonder or excitement in discovery. To make the familiar new is an important skill. A second emotion associated with qualitative research that can benefit from early exposure and practice is getting comfortable with discomfort. Students are instinctively uncomfortable with new spaces and with learning to see and think in ways that are unpracticed. As a result, the discomfort of experiential qualitative research may cause students to reject or try to ignore their own feelings. Exercise 3.2 allows students to experience a space where feelings of discomfort may emerge. However, it also draws attention to the emotion of empathy, which serves as a doorway to understanding and producing "thick description" (Geertz, 1973) that takes into account the inner landscape of participants' feelings.

Classroom Exercise 3.2. The Outsider

GOAL: To describe an unfamiliar place from the point of view of an outsider.

OUTCOMES: This activity helps students understand what it means to experience a place as an outsider. While the exercise can generate excitement because it will be an unfamiliar experience, it can also create a sense of uneasiness and a slight sense of fear of uncertainty, but can help students understand what it means to be the "outsider" in a social group. The advantages and disadvantages of their positionality will also be brought to light.

TIME: 30–60 minutes.

GUIDELINES TO SHARE WITH STUDENTS: Find another site that you have rarely experienced and where you may feel like an outsider. This could be riding on a bus or going to a part of town that you are not used to or going bowling or trying out an activity you have not experienced before. It should involve doing something in a place where you can observe your feelings and experiences while observing others interacting. It is more of a challenge to put yourself in a space where you are interacting with others for the first time. Imagine, for example, that you join a book club where you do not know anyone or no more than one person—the first meeting would be your "outsider" experience. Notice what makes you uncomfortable and why. Examine what questions come to mind when you are in this situation and what focuses your interests. Write as much as you can in a journal about your experiences.

REFLECTION PROMPTS FOR STUDENTS: Read over your journal notes, and using the following prompts, either highlight sections of your journal or write new responses. Share any one or two responses that you find compelling with the whole class or with a small group.

1. Describe the group/activity.
2. Describe your thoughts about the activity or group.
3. What considerations prompted your choice of activity/group?
4. What did it feel like to be an outsider in the group?
5. What felt familiar or strange?
6. Describe the positive and negative feelings that you experienced in this setting. For example, describe the most uncomfortable/comfortable moment you experienced.
7. How did you react to the new group or activity?
8. What did you want/try to do to "fit in"?
9. Did you remember that you are a researcher in this role?
10. What new questions emerged during your experience that surprised you?

Exercises 3.1 and 3.2 can give students glimpses of what is to follow in the course. It connects students to features of qualitative thinking through experiential learning where they come across new questions in familiar and unfamiliar "fields" or spaces. These exercises serve as exemplars of engendering qualitative thinking among students and will initiate questions around observation and the self and other. They will help students to see that being uncomfortable is a good space to be in to observe and learn from participants. Being uncomfortable signals not knowing and helps to bring the researcher to the level of the learner in spaces where others are experts. It initiates an understanding that qualitative data involve coproduction, where the participant (who is the expert on his or her own life experiences) also accedes to the interpretation and understanding of the researcher as the researcher attempts to piece together the different parts of his or her story into a story quilt.

Activities such as these produce a range of experiences for students. Some students may voice their discomfort at being in spaces that make them feel like "outsiders," and may seek to design qualitative research projects that put them in "insider" roles. Although we tackle researcher roles and identities in detail in another chapter, it may help students to contrast the two experiences of Exercises 3.1 and 3.2 to see the advantages and disadvantages of taking on an "insider" or "outsider" position. Educators can share their own experiences of being outsiders in spaces (e.g., being new to the university, being new to higher-education teaching, learning a new skill) and share their reflections of what they learned so that students are less anxious about venturing into research in unknown sites. It may also help students if educators point to the newness and discovery that accompanies such fieldwork so that students start to think about their researcher identity and role.

If experiential learning is one feature of a pedagogy that is holistic, dialogue and role play are other ways of promoting critical thinking and democratic learning. Critical dialogue in classrooms open up spaces for participants to question and explore accepted ideas and beliefs. It implies an openness to rethinking and subjecting assumptions to rounds of questioning. In order to create a space that is conducive to such critical discussion (Giroux, 1985), we have found that an inviting classroom is necessary. Students need to feel safe enough to participate and question freely. As a teacher, this means a commitment to creating an inviting space for students to participate and engage in discussions, listen deeply, and practice tact as an educator when formulating verbal and written responses to students. By tact, we refer to Kingwell's (1995) idea that as educators we need to sometimes curb our desire to express ourselves fully in the classroom. Instead, we need to share space with students so that there is a give-and-take in discussions.

Teaching Qualitative Thinking through Dialogue

Examining assumptions regarding research is one way to begin qualitative thinking. Asking students to write what words come to mind when they hear the word *research* would typically garner responses ranging from Google search engines to interviewing or reading. In order to figure out what assumptions students bring into the classroom about research and what expectations they have regarding learning in research courses, a number of exercises might help to map the terrain. Students influenced by the "smog" of research they have casually encountered over time enter the classroom usually unaware of their own conditioning in the age of "big data." They are used to a survey popping up at various sites they visit, and naturally do not think of research in terms of ethnography or anthropology. While this last is not necessarily a problem, what is problematic is the pervasive idea of evidence as quantitative. Therefore, one of the challenges for teachers of qualitative research is to first understand and then communicate to students the value of and what counts as qualitative evidence.

One of the ways to introduce the idea of what constitutes qualitative evidence is through activities designed to promote critical and divergent thinking. Exercises 3.3 and 3.4 are suggestions for educators to use in classrooms to help students practice thinking qualitatively. They can be used to initiate discussions focused on deepening reflection skills and promoting qualitative thinking.

Classroom Exercise 3.3. 20 Questions

GOAL: To understand and evaluate different types of qualitative evidence and to make questioning a habit of mind (Meier, 2002).

OUTCOMES: At the end of this exercise, students will be able to think about what constitutes different types of qualitative evidence. It encourages them to evaluate, ask questions about evidence, and question their assumptions regarding the nature of evidence. As each group begins to examine the artifacts they have been given, they also embark on a journey of research and socialization into the research process that is both exciting and uncertain. Giving no detailed direction or protocols to students, and instead leaving them with a general idea that they need to come up with questions or themes to explore, puts students in the shoes of researchers.

TIME: 30 minutes.

GUIDELINES FOR THE EDUCATOR: To play the qualitative thinking version of 20 questions, divide students into four or five groups. Give each group a few examples of a specific type of qualitative material. These can range from printed matter, such as magazines, books, and articles, to current or draft sets of field notes from researchers and film documentaries. For example, give four to five contemporary magazines (teen magazines or any magazines targeted at an audience are good choices) to one group; to another group give an excerpt from field notes (perhaps from an ongoing research project that contain possibilities for gender analyses); to a third group give an article's findings on gender play; and to a fourth group, ask that they watch an excerpt from a documentary (e.g., Jhally and Kilbourne's (2010) series *Killing Us Softly*). Pick a theme to make this activity meaningful, fun, and relevant to students.

GUIDELINES TO SHARE WITH STUDENTS: Look at the artifacts you have been given. In your group, brainstorm 20 questions that you think are relevant to the content and form of the artifacts you have in hand. Crystallize into no more than five questions or group into subheadings of no more than five. Present your questions to other groups after a brief explanation of the type of artifact with which you were working.

REFLECTION PROMPTS FOR STUDENTS:

1. Share the process you used to work in your group.
2. How did you examine the artifact and come up with five questions?
3. What assumptions did you make about the artifacts you examined?
4. How would you categorize the questions your group came up with (e.g., content, reflexive, evaluative)?
5. How would you evaluate the artifact you worked with in terms of qualitative evidence?
6. How useful was the artifact in terms of giving you knowledge?
7. What were the limitations of this artifact?
8. What more would you need to know to get more out of these types of data or evidence?
9. What other types of evidence would have helped you?
10. In listening to all groups present their questions, what three themes or questions emerge from the different artifacts?

Classroom exercises such as Exercise 3.3 can facilitate the "wide-awakeness" referred to by Greene (1978), whom we quoted in the beginning of this chapter. These exercises can serve as starting points for questions and for generating topics for research. They can also help students learn to generate questions and make questioning a habit in the research process.

In the next section, we continue the discussion of generating qualitative questions and of creating opportunities for students to engage in asking qualitative questions.

Facilitating Students to Ask Qualitative Questions

There is no disputing that research questions are central to the inquiry process of qualitative research. However, the question that is less easy to answer is—Should research questions be the starting point of research? And if not, what should take its place? Scholars (Hatch, 2002; Metz, 2001) lean in different directions when answering this question. Some, like Metz, assert that the research question is the "starting point and most important issue in developing research" (p. 13). Others, like Hatch, prefer to begin with identifying one's assumptions and belief systems, arguing that beliefs and worldviews have a fundamental impact on the type of research questions posed. Part of the problem is that the process of research, unlike its final presentation, is a messy, nonlinear, and iterative process. Regardless of how one begins, whether with a question or with assumptions, they are both essential to the inquiry process.

Research questions are central to the process and are linked to belief systems and assumptions. Linear thinking does not have a role in this process, as concepts and ideas are constantly shaken up to make room for more connections to occur. Despite this, it is useful to keep in mind the relationship between belief systems and the research question and methodology one chooses.

Critical qualitative researchers, for example, hold questions of power central to their inquiry. The aim of critical research is often to bring about change by examining the processes by which inequities are practiced. Through such change, researchers hope to bring about empowerment and freedom to oppressed groups. Critical qualitative researchers pay attention to what is missing in the scenes they observe and are especially attentive to the politics and power in the situation.

To understand where students at the beginning stages of thinking about qualitative research place themselves within a spectrum of beliefs and methods, we have found it useful to ask them to write a short memo similar to Maxwell's (2008) "researcher identity memo," where students can identify their prior assumptions about the topic and their experiences can influence their approach. In qualitative research, in order to learn qualitative thinking or learn to formulate a research question, it is important to confront what students believe to be true about how the world is ordered, and then ponder different ways of examining the world. A disconnect between knowledge that is usually taken for granted and observed actions can lead to the beginnings of a research project. Qualitative projects can emerge from observations of everyday occurrences.

Qualitative thinking includes an understanding of methodologies, epistemologies, and theories that inform research. Epistemological understanding is possible only if students in the classroom are able to connect such concepts to their own positions and can engage in reflexivity. Questions that are useful prompts for reflexive thinking and for understanding intersubjectivity as the interaction between the researcher's subjectivity and the subjectivity of the participants include:

Why am I thinking this way? Or how did I come to be thinking this way?

What am I taking for granted here?

What do I believe to be true in this situation?

What assumptions do I have about the population I am interested in?

What assumptions do I think this population might have about me?

Do I consider myself an "insider" or "outsider," in relation to this population? Why and in what ways?

These questions prompt a state of continuous reflexivity and may lead one to better formulate the central anchor research questions. The anchor research questions may then address a gap in knowledge or identify where the wrinkles (unwanted or undesired folds) and the creases (intentionally placed demarcations that need to be unpacked or smoothed out) exist in the literature.

In the next section, we offer examples of qualitative thinking from published qualitative works that can illustrate the different ways through which researchers arrive at topics or questions or ways to think about what they observe and what is already known.

Example of Qualitative Thinking Leading to Research from *Sidewalk*

One example of what can spur qualitative thinking can be found in Duneier's (1999) book *Sidewalk*. Dunier saw seemingly homeless men selling books on a New York street and stopped to talk with one of them. He gave the man his card, who remarked that he would put it in his Rolodex. Duneier was intrigued—the homeless man was also apparently an entrepreneur. Duneier's observations and encounter gave rise to a question in his mind: How do these men define and construct their identities? For Duneier, the gap between what he observed and what he understood to be taken for granted—homeless men and entrepreneurship—created a spark of curiosity and questioning that led to his research questions and design. This is an example of how qualitative thinking can arise in the gap between what is observed and what is assumed to be true. In teaching students qualitative research, examples such as these help to illustrate how observation coupled with curiosity can be key to arriving at a research question.

In the next example, a researcher "notices" something taken for granted by everyone else in the research context.

Example of Qualitative Thinking Leading to Research from *Bad Boys*

In *Bad Boys* (2001), Ferguson began as a member of an evaluation team to appraise an intervention for students in an "at-risk" program. When she saw all the students together in a classroom, she realized that all but one was African American and more than 90% were male. This fact disturbed her greatly and even more so when she realized that this was taken for granted by most others at the school, which led her to begin a 3-year participant observation study at the school. Ferguson saw a disturbing fact and wanted to find out more about the race and gender pattern of how these students ended up in the at-risk group. In teaching qualitative research, Ferguson's example serves to remind us that a researcher can arrive at a research question by questioning assumptions at the research site.

Before students can arrive at qualitative research questions, they may need to brainstorm topics for research. While many students have ideas of what they are interested in, the ideas are sometimes either too vague or too specific, neither of which can serve as useful topics for a small-scale course project. To arrive at a project topic, we often suggest that students work in pairs with one student questioning the other on his or her choice of topic.

Reflexive Thinking for Qualitative Research Topics

Research questions may be central to the research process and may emerge from experience, from a suggestion from another researcher, or from a long dialogue with the literature and with peers. In the classroom, for example, trying out this exercise in pairs can generate a deeper understanding of the topic and its significance for the researcher. In Exercise 3.4, students can work in pairs and prompt and critique each other regarding topics suitable for qualitative research projects.

Classroom Exercise 3.4. Brainstorming Qualitative Research Topics

GOAL: Arriving at a research topic that is suitable for qualitative investigation.

OUTCOME: By questioning each other in pairs, students learn to identify suitable research topics that are meaningful to them.

TIME: 20–30 minutes.

GUIDELINES TO SHARE WITH STUDENTS: Write down, in a couple of sentences, your research topic. Share with your partner. Take turns asking each other the following questions regarding your topics for research. Share your thoughts with your partner and give him or her feedback on his or her topic. This exercise uses your self-awareness as a springboard to generate ideas.

1. What about this topic did you find intriguing?
2. What about this topic makes you angry?
3. What about this topic makes you surprised?
4. What about this topic makes you curious to know more?

5. What unanswered questions do you find here?
6. Why is this topic important to you?
7. What qualitative questions can you think of in relation to your project?

REFLECTION PROMPTS FOR STUDENTS:

1. What do you now think about your topic?
2. In what way did the activity help you to understand your topic?
3. In what way is your topic suitable for a qualitative project?

These questions can help students arrive at a deeper understanding of what is important about their topic of interest and can pinpoint areas that can be pursued for a small-scale project. For qualitative projects, we often suggest to students to think of an activity, a place, a group of people, or a process as a way to focus their topics.

In the next section, we move from topic to questions and discuss how students can arrive at a research question that is qualitative.

How to Ask a Qualitative Research Question

Students' early attempts at framing research topics often take the form of problems that need solving rather than issues that need to be explored further. Sometimes their questions are more suited to quantitative research designs—for example, questions comparing two groups or activities and wondering which of the two is better.

Qualitative research questions are generally open-ended, allowing for a multiplicity of findings to emerge. Research questions typically begin with words like *why*, *how*, and *what*. They focus on process or perspectives or place or a group activity. They involve interaction. In Exercise 3.5, we share an activity that can be used by educators to help students represent their research topic in all its complexity and arrive at a question that is researchable. This activity can be redone by students several times and can serve as a graphic representation of the evolution of their thought processes over time. This exercise can be modified and adapted to serve as a reflexive pedagogical device throughout a research project for students and/or faculty examining their own pedagogical thinking about the course. The dialogue will be internal or a dialogue with their journal or perhaps even with other colleagues. The graphic representation can used to "map" the terrain of their own teaching and can serve as a journal of their professional development over time. The activity can be renamed for educators as The Classroom and I (Eye). Inspired by Ellis's (2004) groundbreaking autoethnographic book entitled *The Ethnographic I: A Methodological Novel about Auto-ethnography,* the I and eye are to do with observation, reflection, and reflexivity. In Exercise 3.5, we have made suggestions that educators can use as reflection prompts for their self-development.

Classroom Exercise 3.5. Research Topic and I (Eye)

GOAL: To arrive at a graphic representation of the student's thought processes and connections to the research topic.

OUTCOMES: This exercise is one that students enjoy as they continue modifying the graphic over the semester. As they learn more about their topic and refine their questions, they create newer, and at times more complex, graphics to represent their thinking. This graphic serves as an abstract or a space where everything students are thinking about is represented. By keeping all their efforts in one place, they are also able to trace the development of their own thinking about the research topic and question.

TIME: 1 hour

GUIDELINES TO SHARE WITH STUDENTS: This calls for you to represent your research using the prompts that follow in any visual manner—use a computer or a piece of paper and a pencil or any other means you prefer. After you draw or use the computer to create a diagram representing your topic and position, present your ideas to a small group and come up with questions that may be considered qualitative questions. Present the questions to the class for feedback.

In your graphic representation, be sure to include the following:

1. A topic
2. How you are connected to it.
3. What you want to know about it.
4. The assumptions you have about it, including what you know and do not know.
5. How the topic relates to your own values.
6. How you will go about finding out more.
7. Questions about what you want to know using *what, why,* or *how* as framing strategies.

REFLECTION PROMPTS FOR STUDENTS:

1. What have you learned from this activity?
2. When you look at this activity as a process of thinking, in what way do you anticipate changing this graphic next time?
3. Why was this activity useful/not useful?

Exercise 3.5 helps students to articulate how they are connected to their research. It also helps them to understand and acknowledge their assumptions, how they see the topic, and to arrive at researchable questions. As educators of qualitative researchers, the question that we have often faced in a classroom is how to help students who are steeped in a culture where "data" are synonymous with numbers. Related to this issue, we find that while most students enjoy the classroom exercises, including those that give them a glimpse of fieldwork or engage them in classroom dialogues, there are students who are reluctant to make a shift in their thinking from a quantitative to a qualitative mode, and more often than not, from a postpositivist perspective to an interpretive or critical perspective. In such cases, we have found that peer discussions often are good prompts for helping them reflect, and in other cases, we have stepped in to gently nudge them with questions to try a different perspective. In this and in other chapters, we provide ways in which a holistic approach to teaching qualitative research can help such students become more comfortable with uncertainty and understand the meaning of qualitative evidence.

CHAPTER SUMMARY ● ● ● ● ● ● ● ● ● ● ● ●

In this chapter, we presented a holistic pedagogical approach to teaching qualitative research and in particular, what we termed *qualitative thinking*. We took a pedagogical approach that challenges us to teach with courage—"to be awake and take risks." In addition, we presented different ways that qualitative researchers and faculty have confronted the issue of selecting approaches to use when teaching qualitative inquiry. We also suggested specific activities for the classroom, as well for educators' self-development, that can serve as strategic devices for further dialogue and questioning. The next chapter explores the concepts of bias and positionality and discusses ways to help students increase their abilities to be reflexive.

CHAPTER 4

What Do You Mean That Being "Biased" Isn't Wrong?

Reflexive Exercises to Promote Awareness and Discussion of "Positionality" in Qualitative Research

Often, students are used to attributing a negative connotation to the term *bias,* and an early corrective that teachers of qualitative inquiry sometimes find themselves in the midst of is shifting students' understanding of this term. Rather than seeing it as something to guard against, we need to work on increasing our awareness of our biases and celebrate our "positionality" by way of structured reflexivity exercises. Helping students recognize the impact biases, worldviews, and positionalities have on what (and how) we see and hear, and how they shape our understandings about social realities, prepares them for the self-interrogation that qualitative researchers must engage in continuously. In this context, the role of the researcher as insider, outsider, friend and peer, and companion, among others, is examined. In addition, the issues surrounding empathic listening as an empowering or silencing effect is also discussed within the context of critical research. If research has social justice or empowerment goals, what role does bias play in such contexts? We explore and discuss alternative ways of conceptualizing and teaching empathic listening.

In this chapter, we:

- Unpack bias and positionality as central organizing concepts for novice researchers.
- Provide exercises to increase awareness and understanding about how to develop a reflexive thinking process.
- Review ways to approach the introduction of ethics discussions related to human subjects research.

Discussing and Tackling the Questions of Bias

Postpositivist thinking and training has ingrained in students and researchers the idea that impersonal and neutral detachment make for good research. In this paradigm, bias and subjectivity are regarded as unscientific and the personal a distraction and problem to objectivity.

In qualitative research, questions of subjectivity and bias come up often since the researcher is the instrument of research. In other words, it is the researcher who designs the study, gathers the data, interprets the data for findings or themes, and presents the results. Researchers respond to environmental cues, perceive situations holistically, describe nonverbal information, and explore the unexpected—they appreciate context rather than trying to control it. Qualitative researchers have discussed ways to transcend bias. One of the most accepted ways to take steps to reduce bias is to increase the time spent in the "field" or with participants. Another way has been through a review of data by peers. A "critical friends" approach of peer debriefing has also been used where peers look for and ask questions that trigger an awareness of blind spots or omissions. Allowing other researchers or assistants to gather data has been another way in which qualitative researchers have tackled the issue of bias. In addition, accounts from participants are used to supplement researcher-gathered data. This is often termed *respondent validation* (Hammersley & Atkinson, 1993). Journaling or noting one's thoughts and assumptions prior to beginning a study has been used by qualitative researchers to become aware of any biases with which they might enter the field. One way to figure out and become aware of one's assumptions is by "interviewing the investigator" (Chenail, 2011). This allows the researcher to modify interviews or protocols before going into the field.

Another way that qualitative researchers have adopted to minimize bias has been to incorporate participant voices in the analysis and writing of research, a point that has been critiqued by critical qualitative researchers.

What Is Bias in Critical Qualitative Research?

Critical qualitative research challenges the neutrality of research and further challenges the ways in which the question of bias is tackled, even by qualitative researchers. Morse (2003) argues that qualitative researchers attempting to overcome bias may end up with results that are weak and general without generating new insights into the phenomenon of investigation. In qualitative research, bias is often regarded as a problem of representation. Novice researchers, in an attempt to overcome bias, may inadvertently weaken the design and intention of the research. For example, as Morse (2003) notes, "biasphobia" results in an attempt to circumvent what researchers regard as bias in selection. In the process, qualitative researchers can make the mistake of attempting to diversify representation through sampling. In choosing people to represent the larger population—for example, participants from different ethnic groups—an equitable representation may be misleading if the phenomenon under investigation occurs more often or robustly within one ethnic population or gender. Similarly, Woodley and Lockard (2016) argue that while snowball sampling may be thought of as leading to a sample that is restricted through limited networks, they nevertheless advocate for snowball sampling. They argue that snowball sampling is a way to get at hard-to-reach, hidden populations or marginalized groups. Not only can snowball sampling access these populations and groups, in addition, they can also serve as a way to understand networks and social circles (Heckathorn, 2011), even if the sample sizes are small. While snowball sampling is often taken to mean accessing one participant who will then open the door to others, in reality, snowball sampling requires casting a wide net through word of mouth or via the Internet and Facebook (Baltar & Brunet, 2012) in a variety of spaces (Woodley & Lockard, 2016). Daly and Lumley (2002) offer a similar perspective when they describe a process for selection in qualitative research. Even if the sample size is small, they advocate a purposeful sample where the experience is strongest felt. Within the participant group, in many cases, it is likely that different opinions and perspectives will be present, which can then lead the researcher to go back to the field and enlarge the sample size to find participants who experience that difference. An additional rationale in favor of snowball sampling is its potential to understand networks. Since hidden populations often develop networks that work in confidence and confidentiality, snowball sampling gets at social and interactional circles that can lead to a deeper theoretical understanding and generate new insights.

In qualitative research, depth in understanding is the goal since if findings merely document learning what "I already knew or my grandmother knew," it means that inadequate data were gathered and the data were not deep enough or the analysis lacked complexity and nuances.

Morse's (2003) advice in *Biasphobia* is one that we advocate in teaching the meanings of bias in qualitative research. Rather than seek to avoid bias, it is better to confront and even embrace bias. By this we mean it is important to understand what students mean by bias, what the difference is between bias and worldview and positionality, and how the three might be interwoven in different ways. The lesson to learn in the selection of participants is to find those participants who are most engaged with the phenomenon or activity one is interested in, rather than find people from different groups who may be marginally engaged in the activity. It is the activity or phenomenon and its engagement that will yield a thorough understanding and new insights that can then be explored with different groups later.

Critical qualitative researchers point out that typical ways of attempting to transcend bias in qualitative research by including the voices of participants or respondents in the analysis may result in appropriating the voices of "others" in which patterns of domination are reinforced and not challenged. According to Smith (1988), researchers can adopt a stance of intimidation, ingratiation, self-promotion, or supplication. Of these, again according to Smith (1988), supplication is the means by which the researcher accepts and acknowledges his or her reliance on the knowledge and expertise of the researched for guidance. While the attempt is toward reciprocal power relations, the responsibility for the final product or text, as some qualitative feminist researchers have pointed out, continues to be problematic since it is not merely the politics of visibility that one is contending with but also the politics of representation. Researchers need to take responsibility for the unequal power relations. Power may be shared—however, it is questioned by some scholars whether it is desirable to share the responsibility for the research with participants who were not involved in conceptualizing the research or its design. The reflexivity of the researcher is one of the most accepted ways to transcend bias in qualitative research.

What Is Positionality and How Does It Influence Qualitative Research Projects?

Positionality is the acknowledgment that a researcher is positioned by gender, class, race, age, sexuality, ethnicity, language, culture, and biography. The qualitative researcher needs to become aware that all of these may either enhance or inhibit some insights on the part of the researcher. Banks (1998) argued that it was important to uncover the values that underpin social science research. He said, "I now believe that the biographical journeys of researchers greatly influence their values, their research questions and the knowledge they construct" (p. 4). He went on to point out that what is visible in disseminated research is construed as the product of researchers' minds while their beliefs and values are largely muted. Banks was referring to the issues that were later raised by feminists, womanists, and ethnic studies scholars who supported the view that a researcher's belief system and political and social standpoint would influence the type of research he or she conducted and how the researcher conducted it. In other words, situationality and positionality—the context or where the researcher was from and where he or she was located—were equally important to reflect on in learning to do research as much as it was important to understand society.

In qualitative research, learning about one's positionality takes place over the course of the research, and reflexivity is the guiding tool to remain aware of in the process. Reflexivity is the process by which a researcher remains aware of his or her contexts and circumstances, and his or her location and relational power. Teaching and learning about reflexivity is central to qualitative research. There are many ways in which to teach students to develop reflexivity and several classroom activities to try with students to promote and grow reflexivity. Qualitative researchers need to "acquire the habit of viewing" (Gouldner, 1970, p. 490) their own beliefs and worldviews as much as they observe and document the beliefs and perspectives of research participants. The "habit of viewing" means learning to be aware of their own attitudes and perspectives toward a variety of events or circumstances, and how their focus is affected by where they are from and by their own biographies.

Kaufman (2013) suggests growing reflexivity through classroom activities that are writing based. He describes an activity that simulates peer discussions in a safe environment by asking students to write and comment on one another's thoughts and reflections on a series of prompts presented by the instructor that are chosen according to the course being taught. Students each pass a piece of paper on which their thoughts are written to the person next to them and continue to pass the papers and write their own comments on the papers so that in the end, there are a series of comments on every reflection.

Teaching reflexivity to qualitative researchers can be modeled by instructors by sharing their own reflexivity regarding their positionality with the students. This is perhaps the most memorable way students begin to understand what this process might look like and the overall importance it plays within qualitative inquiry projects. Teaching reflexivity to students in a single teaching module, as you might assume, may not achieve the results an instructor wants. For example, Sargeant (2012) described her experience of teaching reflexivity to students who did not produce assessments of their own roles in their research projects. Instead, they had drifted to discussions that were more general. Sargeant concluded that it was necessary to build reflective practice into the entire course rather than teach it as a separate unit, particularly if students did not have enough practice with reflection.

Reflexivity is not a task—it is an ongoing process—it is an epistemology. And helping students understand the very nature of reflexivity processes is often at the heart of what faculty are doing at all levels of their teaching when they incrementally assist students into this way of knowing.

Hierarchical Positionings and the "Other" in Qualitative Research

Critical qualitative researchers centralize power relations between the researcher and the researched and attempt to confront and minimize that hierarchical positioning. However, they are aware that despite everything, the researcher still had advantages that are denied to the researched. An example is that of fieldwork. Despite all attempts made by the researcher to assure the participants that leaving the research will not be detrimental to their interests, it is nevertheless also true that often in fieldwork settings, when the researcher enters a network of relationships, it is far easier for the researcher to leave these settings and relationships than it is for the research respondents to do so.

The Role of the Qualitative Researcher

Ethical Considerations

Teaching novice researchers about the necessity of expanding their ethical considerations is essential, and pedagogical decisions related to this area are deserving of careful attention. A common starting point is to work with students through the IRB at your home institution, including exposing them to the Collaborative Institutional Training Initiative (CITI) and their certification process or parallel training offered by your institution. The CITI materials can be very useful to guide in-class discussions. They can be used to help demystify research processes that interface with human beings as well as reinscribe the practices that can minimize risk and maintain integrity within the consenting process. Some faculty have partnered with members of the IRB and invited them in for a class presentation or workshop. Others may opt for sharing examples of IRB-approved protocols. Asking students to carefully examine in small groups the phrasing used to communicate the specific steps taken to minimize risk and increasing procedural transparency are often quite fruitful. Facilitating this discussion so that it also addresses the ways researchers need to be patient and resilient while crafting the data collection procedures, including access to the population they wish to sample, as well as plans for safe storage and eventual destruction of raw data to help ensure confidentiality, is of paramount importance.

Inevitably, these classroom discussions come in layers and need to be partially repeated throughout the course so that students understand that with each stage of research there are important ethical considerations to be examined. All researchers can benefit from intentional conversations with trusted and qualified peers to help mull over the ethical dilemmas that may arise at any time throughout the process of conducting research. It is important that students know that the larger community of researchers are bound to one another within the pursuit of this level of integrity, and the concept of peer review, while important in all areas of research, takes on an additional level of significance in the area of ethics. Helping students practice discernment and interpretation, as they discuss ethical case scenarios, for example, serves not only the individual novice researcher but also has the potential to strengthen the practices of the overall research community.

Outsider, Insider, Friend, Peer, Companion

Qualitative researchers can play several roles while conducting research and analysis. The role of the researcher, whether it be that of a friend, insider, or outsider, can be more fluid than fixed and may change over time in the field. All the roles present possibilities for respectful interactions with the participants. Outsider researchers prepare to enter the field while insider researchers need a different type of preparation to help them navigate the self and the participants. *Insiders* and *outsiders* are broad terms that can contain within them more definitive relations like friends or peers or colleagues or "companions" (Bourdieu & Wacquant, 1992).

Insider research is conducted by researchers who are also members of the community in which they are conducting research. Researchers conducting "insider" research has increased recently with more novice researchers undertaking practitioner inquiry or inquiry within their own settings as part of action research. Both action research and autoethnographies call for insider research and researchers explain their own positionality as part of the research. While some scholars define insiders as researchers who study a social group to which they belong, (Loxley & Seery, 2008; Naples, 2003), others have pointed out that having a priori knowledge of a group without necessarily being a member was enough to be regarded as an insider (Hellawell, 2006).

Some scholars (Banks, 1998; Merton, 1972) rejected the insider–outsider arguments that claimed superior positionality for either position. Insiders often claimed that only insiders could research culture because as a member of the group, they could understand it and have unique insights into it. Outsiders similarly claimed that outsiders could accurately describe the culture and interactions without being clouded by prior judgment. Merton argued that both points of view were needed in social science research and declared that depending on the context, we are all both insiders and outsiders. Perhaps the best way to consider these roles is to view them as being on a continuum rather than as fixed positions with no relation to each other.

While there are multiple definitions of what it means to be an insider or an outsider in research and variations and subcategories— for example, "external insider" or "internal outsider" (Banks, 1998) or total or partial insider (Chavez, 2008)—the real issues with being an insider or outsider is learning to navigate one's positionality while negotiating trust with the participants.

Reflexivity prior to entering the field for research may require researchers to think about where they stand with regard to the research project prior to entering the field. The reflexive activity in Exercise 4.1 might help the researcher to prepare him- or herself to enter the field.

Classroom Exercise 4.1. Teaching Reflexivity

GOAL: To prepare oneself to start research and understand the roles that one can take on in the field.

OUTCOMES: This activity helps students understand and reflect on what they already know about the participants, the context, and the research site. It can help students to become aware of their own preconceived ideas regarding the research topic and the participants. The activity can also help students to imagine themselves in interaction with participants, what to anticipate, and to become more aware of their preconceived ideas regarding "bias" and their identities.

TIME: 1 hour.

GUIDELINES TO SHARE WITH STUDENTS: Students should spend 10–15 minutes answering the following:

1. What are you familiar with at the research site?
2. What do you already know about the people?
3. How do people respond to you at the site?
4. How do you anticipate the group you are researching will respond to you?
5. What do you anticipate learning that you do not already know?
6. What are some things you will need to navigate or work on to be able to conduct your research?
7. Pick the role or combination of roles that you consider will be most

appropriate for you in the field at least in the beginning of the research (e.g., insider, outsider, friend, peer, companion).

After everyone completes his or her writing, exchange notes with a partner. Your partner will read the notes and follow up with the following questions to aid reflexivity. Look at the questions and modify them as appropriate to the roles that your partner has written about. Take turns asking each other the questions.

1. Given the familiarity/unfamiliarity with the site and people, what advantages does it give you as a researcher in conducting your research?

   Follow-up prompts:
   - Historical background.
   - Nonverbal cues.
   - Not seen as an outsider and therefore can blend into the setting.
   - Prior knowledge of how to approach different people in the context.

2. Given the familiarity/unfamiliarity of the research site and people, how does this knowledge disadvantage you as a researcher?

   Follow-up prompts:
   - Preexisting tensions can influence who participates and who is not approached.
   - Unable to get good examples and explanations because of an assumed overfamiliarity with the context.
   - Unable to get good examples or rapport because of distance from particular members of the group.
   - Unable to gain trust because one is seen as partial to a particular viewpoint.
   - Perhaps too invested in some ideas at the site and therefore not seeking out diverse points of view.

REFLECTION PROMPTS FOR STUDENTS: After students have completed their exercise and dialogue activity, debrief with the following questions to help them reflect on their activity.

1. How did this exercise help you learn about the ways in which you can prepare to enter the field?

2. How will you "manage impressions" (Goffman, 1959) in the field?

3. How did your discussion with your partner help you think about the ways in which "shape shifting" or "skin walking" (i.e., moving from one shape into another) was a good metaphor for changing roles in the field?

4. What are the ways in which you anticipate "shape shifting" in the field?

5. How do you now anticipate participants changing their roles in response to the research you are conducting? For example, is it possible for a friend to now become a friend–informant (Taylor, 2011)?

6. How will these changes affect your power relations with participants?

Identity and the Qualitative Researcher

Students in doctoral programs develop their identities as scholars and researchers over the course of their study. Helping students to become increasingly reflexive also includes providing them with opportunities to increase their listening skills and work toward higher degrees of empathy. These are aspects of building their researcher identity, a central concept that permeates throughout all pedagogical activities designed to help novice researchers. Kamler and Thomson (2008) argued the following: "doctoral writing is best understood as text work/identity work. By this we mean that texts and identities are formed together, in, and through writing. The practices of doctoral writing simultaneously produce not only a dissertation but also a doctoral scholar"(p. 508). Exercise 4.2 can help students think about their positionality and identity in thoughtful ways.

Classroom Exercise 4.2. Understanding Your Positionality

GOAL: Students reflect on positionality and identity.

OUTCOME: Students learn to be deliberately aware of what influences the way they think.

TIME: 15 minutes, plus 15 minutes for debriefing.

GUIDELINES TO SHARE WITH STUDENTS: Write your thoughts about the following on an index card:

- How do I describe myself? What identity markers do I use?
- What shapes my perspectives?
- How do I perceive the people around me?
- What shapes my worldview?

GUIDELINES FOR REFLECTION AND DISCUSSION WITH STUDENTS: Share your comments with your peers in a small group.

- How does identity affect the way we perceive, know, or experience the world?
- How is positionality related to identity?
- How can empathy help with your perceptions and experiences?
- How does this positionality and identity exercise help you think about the participants in your research?

This activity allows students to examine their own awareness of their identity as it relates to the ways in which they are socialized to think or perceive. It draws awareness to habitual patterns of perception based on taken-for-granted ways of thinking or being. It draws attention to the need to become more mindful in the research process.

CHAPTER SUMMARY ● ● ● ● ● ● ● ● ● ● ● ● ●

Overall, this chapter provided several ways to consider how to approach teaching the concept of reflexivity and designing ways to help students increase their sensibilities toward qualitative inquiry work including ethical considerations. The next chapter entertains ways to assist students with crafting a meaningful research problem.

CHAPTER 5

Crafting a Research Problem
The "So What?" Question

Teaching students to craft a research problem and distinguish between a research problem and a practical problem is one of the foundations of a research course.

In this chapter, we offer:

- Practical pointers on how to approach this topic as well as suggestions for readings that faculty can use to plan their teaching module on this unit.

- Ways to assist students with understanding the nature of a research problem and how to craft a "problem statement."

- A review of seminal qualitative research works as an exemplar of what researchers mean when they say they have identified a "gap" in the literature.

- A discussion of the way researchers build a convincing rationale for why a research problem ought to be further examined by way of empirical research.

- Suggestions for the use of peer critique or peer review.

The "So What?" Question

Research is a mysterious adventure that inspires passion
and holds many surprises.
—UMBERTO ECO (2015, p. xxvi)

Eco (2015) conveys the essence of what research can be; more than mere procedure, it is an exploration and discovery that can be exciting and requires training that can cultivate the research imagination. The "so what?" question in qualitative research is often considered at the beginning—during the crafting of the research question. Why is this research necessary? What do we need to learn and understand that we did not know before? These questions need to be asked at every stage of the research process to yield deeper thinking about the research focus, the process, and the analysis. Polkinghorne (2006) argues that students in qualitative research methods courses are quicker to pick up the procedural aspects of methods than the interpretive skills. A course that emphasizes procedures and the how-tos is a carryover from the influences of quantitative research where method-driven research ensures objectivity (Polkinghorne, 2006). Perception, reasoning, interpretation, and storytelling—all features of qualitative research—require the development and practice of a set of creative and intellectual processes that are in line with the researcher being the instrument of research. A teacher of qualitative research, therefore, has the responsibility of nurturing the imagination alongside the logical reasoning to socialize qualitative researchers.

Students' Responses to Research Methods Courses

Studies on students' responses to research methods courses report that students, prior to taking a course, are generally anxious and worry that they may not possess the necessary skill level to succeed. Although much of the empirical research on student attitudes toward research methods courses (Kain, Buchanan, & Mack, 2001; Spalter-Roth & Van Vooren, 2008) use surveys and are broad based in terms of target audiences (including undergraduates and quantitative and qualitative courses), it is nevertheless a reminder to us as faculty teaching these courses that students' initial dispositions need to be considered in our teaching. In terms of teaching students how to think of a research question and work out a research problem, it may be a good idea to start with students' views of what they think this is about. Exercise 5.1 provides a few preliminary questions that can serve as a warm-up exercise for this topic and start a dialogue.

Classroom Exercise 5.1. Opening a Conversation

GOAL: Getting warmed up to learning research methods.

OUTCOMES: Students can get a sense of what they already know about research methods and the assumptions they hold about what skills and dispositions they need in order to grow into researchers.

Time: 20–30 minutes.

Guidelines for the educator: Distribute index cards and have students answer the following questions:

1. What was the last research methods class you took and when?
2. What are three skills you think are most important for qualitative researchers?
3. What skills, knowledge, or dispositions do you think you need to learn to be a good qualitative researcher?

After students spend about 10 minutes answering the questions, they can share with the class what they wrote. The main points can be summarized and projected to the class. This activity allows students to think about what knowledge they already possess. In addition, some of the skills for qualitative research can be mentioned if they were not brought up by the students, such as curiosity, empathy, attentiveness, and reflexivity, and directly relating to the researcher as the instrument of research, a point that students need to understand in depth over the course of the class.

Qualitative pedagogy has drawn from experiential learning and reflection so that the student is at the center—it is the student who experiences, learns from, and reflects on the experience, asks more questions, and perhaps goes back into the field. Experiential learning is drawn from the work of Dewey (1938) and Kolb and Kolb (2012), who advocate experience as a key component of learning that allows for reflection. Reflection is a core construct of qualitative research and the attendant reflexivity concept goes in depth so that researchers can see and question why and what they see. Examining assumptions is necessary for students to start thinking about why their research is significant and why they need to think about the "so what?" aspect of their research. Exercise 5.2 can be used in class for examining prior assumptions regarding research.

Classroom Exercise 5.2. Examining Assumptions

Goal: Learning to practice reflexivity through examining one's own assumptions.

Outcome: To help students understand that one has assumptions that need unpacking regarding all aspects of research.

Time: 20 minutes.

Guidelines for the educator: Pick a topic that provokes diverse opinions, such as obesity, school choice, or poverty. Ask students to write down one sentence about the topic and share with a small group. Then have students reflect on where their assumptions or ideas come from (experiences, reading, what people say . . . , etc.).

REFLECTION PROMPTS FOR STUDENTS:

1. Share what you have written with others in your group. Read everyone's responses.
2. What responses did you see everyone has in common?
3. What was different?
4. Share why you have these ideas about the topic. Where do you think you obtained these ideas?

At the end of the activity, lead a debriefing session with students. Ask them, for example:

1. What did you learn from this activity?
2. How did the activity make you feel?

Exercise 5.2 allows students to see that there are many assumptions that we carry around about everyday life that need to be examined and unpacked when conducting research. It can be a segue to introduce them to the concept of Bourdieu and Wacquant's (1992) "habitus" as a way of understanding and linking the many impressions, beliefs, and values that we carry around and that accrue over time and become concretized into "This is how we do things." However, unpacking these assumptions can also be difficult for students and can create some degree of discomfort. The debriefing session can be used to explain to students that habitus cannot be changed overnight and that awareness of one's assumptions is the goal for qualitative research. Also, a habit of awareness is possible only if one asks questions of oneself.

A second activity that can be used for the same purpose but at a more personalized level is asking students to write a mini-autobiography of issues that have affected or shaped their belief and values. If they are asked to add into their experiences in the social context, it can link issues that are going on in society with their personal beliefs and vice versa. This can be a three-part activity:

- The first part is to ask students to write a short autobiography that links multiple contexts (e.g., home, school, society) to how they shaped their own beliefs and values or their decisions regarding education and career.
- The second part of this activity is to ask students to share their autobiographies with another person in the class.
- The third part is a debriefing dialogue in class about what students learned from the exercise.

Exercise 5.3 encourages students to examine assumptions made between personal and political research.

Classroom Exercise 5.3. Examining Assumptions through Autobiographical Writing

GOAL: Connecting the "personal with the political."

OUTCOMES: Students learn that issues they are most passionate about often have an autobiographical link and that research often links the personal and the political.

TIME: 20 minutes.

GUIDELINES FOR THE EDUCATOR: Ask students the following questions as prompts for discussion:

1. What did you learn from writing this particular autobiography?
2. What did you find most difficult? Why?
3. What surprised you during the process? Why?
4. What influences coalesced to create your own set of values or assumptions regarding education, career, or other strong beliefs you might have?

Like Exercise 5.2, Exercise 5.3 leads students into a "habit" of reflecting on and being aware of their previously held assumptions. These are useful and crucial skills for novice researchers to learn and practice.

What Is a Research Problem in Qualitative Research?

This question often causes confusion among students in no small part because of the way they have been socialized to think about the word *problem* with only a negative connotation. Recasting the word *problem* as a puzzle, curiosity, or site for inquiry in addition to something that causes frustration, alarm, consternation, or harm can often be a good place to start.

Second, "research problems" are generally connected, or linked, to prior problems rather than disconnected. Therefore, this requires reading and comprehension of the literature to best understand some aspect of these connections before crafting a statement about a particular research problem one wishes to investigate. And third, the process of problem setting, or problem creation, is essentially a process of generating questions within the context of what the existing literature offers, how it can prod researchers forward, and how a sophisticated literature review can signify "gaps" or silences in meaning and/or implications. Problem setting often has to do with learning to problematize familiar issues so that new questions can be asked of existing phenomena. A problem or issue becomes researchable once one learns to problematize. In other words, the ability to figure out what question to ask about an existing phenomenon, dig deeper, and introduce complexity all make for researchable problems. For example, if in one school there is apparently a narrow gap between the achievement of students from wealthy and poor backgrounds, it may yield several questions that can be researched:

> Why does this school succeed where many others do not?
>
> Who is responsible for the success?
>
> What is responsible for the success?
>
> To what degree does a sense of belonging play into students' success in school?

Similarly, if a school has a consistently high turnover of principals, several questions may be asked that might overturn taken-for-granted explanations of the reasons for such turnover:

> What is the effect of the turnover on climate, teacher morale, and student success?
>
> What are teachers' and parents' perspectives of the school and the leadership of the school?
>
> And most important, what are the last three principals' perceptions and experiences of turnover in the school?

From these questions, more might emerge and a rationale for conducting the research can be constructed. A rationale for a study is nested within a selective, critical reading of the literature.

Designing ways to facilitate students' interaction with these elements of understanding and developing research problem statements lead to more effectively designed research questions. Learning to widen and deepen novice researchers' understandings of the various types of questions involved in a qualitative study will help to elevate the overall quality of the project. For example, assisting novice researchers with distinguishing between researchable problems and practical problems can quickly reveal the cognitive dissonance that results when trying to engage in this type of inquiry thinking.

Distinguishing between Researchable Problems and Practical Problems

Finding issues or questions in qualitative research involves finding researchable problems or questions that can be answered through research. In qualitative research, students are often directed toward a topic of interest that is then focused on and leads to a researchable question. Since students are often thinking about how they use research in their everyday experience—in other words, even if it is to buy a new car or look for the right school for their child—it requires some amount of digging and familiarizing oneself with the options and the data. These are practical issues and problems to which students apply their skills of information gathering on an everyday basis. In qualitative research, they bring these rather well-developed skills that are also limiting to some extent. They might expect quick results, whereas in research contexts the researchable problem is not only going to take some time to refine the issue, question, or problem but it is also going to take significant time in the field to answer.

One way to begin finding and refining a research issue or finding a purpose to the research might be to start with the action. Some scholars advocate going into a field and figuring out what in a particular context might be important to research. This means doing some preliminary fieldwork with the goal of understanding a context, an environment, and determining what is uppermost on the minds of the people in the field. This may change over time. For example, one of us went into a school in order to research innovative alternative schools and how schools practice innovations, to find that the school was engaged in a debate and battles around democratic governance, freedom, and community among the teachers. Therefore, the research focus on innovations was put on hold while the much more immediate question of how schools practice and negotiate the twin challenges of democracy and community was investigated instead.

What Makes a Problem Researchable?

Most students begin by asking questions or coming up with topics that are either too broad or too narrow. Showing students some examples of how research questions can be too broad or too narrow allows them to understand the difference and to also accept that it may take a few tries to get the research question right. One common error that comes up with an emphasis on the "research problem" is that the purpose of the research, which is connected closely to the research problem itself, can get deflected. When it comes to creating a rationale for research, it is important for students to create a rationale for the purpose of their research, rather than focusing solely on the significance of the research problem. In other words, the research problem serves as the background for the topic. Problematizing the issues raised and critically reviewing the existing solutions to the problem can lead to a "gap" or an omission or a facet not yet explored. The purpose of the research shows why the new research is needed.

Researchable problems are those that have significance, that can add some new knowledge to what we already know, and investigate aspects of issues that have been ignored. Researchable problems need to be doable and time bound. While research can continuously reveal more issues that need to be investigated, it is important for students to create a boundary around their research. What time, space, and other forms of restrictions can they draw around their research that can allow for it to be doable? In Exercise 5.4, students can practice presenting research problems that then lead to the research questions.

Classroom Exercise 5.4. Linking Qualitative Questions and Research Purpose

The previous chapters have discussed how instructors can facilitate students to ask qualitative questions. In this activity, students are asked to explain and present their research question framed within a research problem or issue and discuss the purpose of their research.

GOAL: Learn to articulate the purpose and rationale of the study by situating it within a research issue.

OUTCOMES: Students will formulate a logical argument for their study and present it to their peers. Students will offer critical, constructive feedback to their peers.

TIME: The activity should take approximately 6 minutes for each person, including time for changeovers. No student should present for more than 4 minutes. Doing this activity in small groups will cut down the time considerably.

GUIDELINES TO SHARE WITH STUDENTS: Think about your research project and in a few lines on an index card, note the following:

1. What is your qualitative question?
2. What is the purpose of your study?
3. What is your rationale? Why does this study matter?

After writing these notes, look at them and practice in your mind how you can communicate your study and its purpose in a few minutes to the class or a group.

GUIDELINES FOR THE EDUCATOR: Introduce this activity by asking students to imagine that they are at a party or a family gathering when someone comes along and says, "I hear you are doing a research study. What is it about?" In addition, ask students to look up or show them a couple of vignettes from the "Three Minute Thesis" website (*http://threeminutethesis.org*), where they can see some examples of presentations. While the Three Minute Thesis presentations are quite formal, it can teach students to formulate an argument and rationale for their study.

Next, ask students to either get into small groups or talk to the whole class about their research idea and topic. Peers can give feedback on sheets of paper via questions, comments, or suggestions.

REFLECTION PROMPTS FOR STUDENTS: Take a few minutes to read the comments, questions, and suggestions handed in by your peers. Make a note of a few points regarding the following questions and share with your peers:

1. What did you learn about your research as you were trying to formulate your talk?
2. What did the comments from your peers teach you or inspire you to consider that you had not considered before?

This activity requires students to go deeper into their research question and learn to formulate an argument or rationale for their study that is grounded within a context.

Advocacy Research

Advocacy research often begins with a practical problem that requires research and generates answers that in turn solves problems. Such practical problems are not the one-time look-up issues of where to find resources but are more in-depth issues regarding communication or collaboration or community problems involving multiple players and issues. Advocacy research has to do with advocating for a particular cause or fighting injustice or seeking a community-based solution to a problem identified by the community. In this sense, advocacy research is collaborative, emerges from a cooperative alliance with the community, and brings in the community as coresearchers. The goal of advocacy research is usually specific and driven by the needs of the community. As students make decisions about what type of research they are planning to do, the exercises in this chapter help them think through their stances with respect to research design, research rationale, and collaboration. By considering all of these, students begin to be aware of how their own identities begin to take shape as graduate or doctoral students and as emerging scholars and researchers. As mentioned in other chapters, the researcher identity is an integral part of finding a focus and crafting a research question.

Identity Work and the Research Question

The researcher enters the field with assumptions, values, beliefs, and dispositions. All of these make up a particular researcher identity— however, a researcher's identity is not a fixed entity or predetermined. Instead, it emerges from a continuous process of learning and reflection and adapts and grows as new learning occurs. While there are many theories of identity formation that can inform this discussion, in teaching students about what identity formation is and how a researcher identity is continuously crafted, we suggest two theories that can help illustrate the concept. The postmodern theory of a fluid identity can be explained alongside critical theory that promotes a reflective self. The postmodern fluid identity looks at the ways in which a researcher identity is not fixed and instead is constantly negotiated and constructed. It is a continuous process that takes into account the researcher's way of knowing, the agency of the researcher at any given time, and the ongoing negotiation of relationships with participants. In this sense, the researcher is like a companion in the research, present and negotiating his or her identity in relation to the participants and sites. Critical self-reflection promotes an awareness of self. The goal of self-reflection is to become completely aware of the power, privileges, and status of one's identity in relation to the world around us and in relation to the participants. As an iterative process, critical self-reflection strives to understand the positionality of the researcher at any given time. Both ways of thinking about researcher identity acknowledge that the researcher needs to continuously be aware of researcher identity and what goes into its makeup. The researcher enters the field with a particular identity that is made up of assumptions, values, beliefs, and dispositions. These are repeatedly reflected on as lessons are absorbed in the field. Each role or way in which a researcher identity is imagined can also be seen as a subjective site where reflexivity and awareness can grow. To start with the process of understanding researcher identity, a classroom exercise that brings it to the forefront can help.

Researcher identity can be linked to how researchers see their roles. Exercise 5.5 allows students to brainstorm how different roles and identity hats can perhaps lead to different ways in which they approach the field and their research.

Classroom Exercise 5.5. Imagining Researcher Roles and Identity

GOAL: Helping students see that the researcher role is multifaceted and not limited.

OUTCOMES: Students will see that as researchers, imagining several roles can be a creative way to conduct research; additionally, it can also help students see the field in a variety of ways.

TIME: 40 minutes.

GUIDELINES FOR THE EDUCATOR: Lead a brainstorming activity by asking students:

"What are the different ways in which you can imagine yourself in the field? As an example, 'A researcher can be like a detective. . . .'"

After students have come up with several responses, share Table 5.1 with the students and have them fill it out with their own ideas.

Each imaginative role can be seen as a site of subjectivity with the possibility for increased researcher awareness by way of incrementally more complex reflexivity exercises.

Asking the "So What?" Question

The "so what?" question is a shorthand way of prodding the researcher at the very earliest stages of the research project to wonder about who the reading audiences might be for the results of the study. This is the beginning of the "Implications" section of the written research report. Students can initially be put off or offended when they hear faculty use this often asked question, "So what?" because some students hear this question as implying their study isn't important and no one will care about it. It can strike at the core of their doubt about being able to be a researcher, yet this is a necessary growing pain for novice researchers. The pedagogical empathy required at this moment often helps determine the student's overall attitude toward doubt and ambiguity that are ever present during various stages of conducting research. In fact, in order to build and nurture curiosity within novice researchers, particular exercises can be developed to help them embrace doubt and ambiguity as positive experiences as researchers rather than live within the negative connotations of these concepts.

TABLE 5.1. Imagining the Researcher

A researcher is like a . . .	What activities does this entail?	How does this influence my disposition?	How does this play out in my own research project?
Detective	Investigating how something happened, looking for clues, and interviewing main participants.	I may be regarded as a bit of an outsider, with a job to do. But I am interested in finding out all aspects of the issue.	In my project, I find that the role of detective plays out in terms of finding the history of the way in which power has been shared among teachers over time so that it has now become part of the culture.
Journalist	I am looking to find out all the main participants at the site. Who can give me access and to what? I want to hear from all participants.	Participants may think I am here just to get my own work done, as in doing my research for a publication. But I am interested in telling the story of the participants and of this site so that everyone knows about it.	I find that thinking like a journalist has helped me to uncover the history of this project, which has in turn helped with a clearer understanding of the issues involved.
Change agent	I am here to ensure that the current problems are examined and resolved.	I am interested in the problem and am interested in resolution and action. I am not here to simply gather narratives but to see participants enact change.	My presence here seems to have influenced some people into taking action. Is this research advocacy research?

Consultant	I am here to help and serve as a critical eye or give advice.
Catalyst	My presence causes people to reflect and think differently about their problems.
Collaborator	I am part of the community and their partner.
Ghostly interlocutor	I am here to tell the story of the participants. They tell the stories and I simply narrate them. I am the ghostly interlocutor in the narrative.
Critical friend	I serve as the critical eye for the group. I can see what is going on as if standing on the boundary of the outsider/insider.
Companion	I am here as a traveling companion—for the journey.

Novice researchers can be doubly helped at this juncture if they can transfer the "so what?" question from their own study ideas to using it to build their critical eye when reviewing the literature. The next section specifically addresses exercises to help sharpen novice researchers' abilities to critically read and review the literature with an eye toward finding the gap. Gaps in the literature sometimes can be present because the research community has collectively taken a leap of faith or a leap in logic or neglected possible implications of the current collective research findings regarding a particular topic. New studies of significance can be formed within the gap.

Identifying the "So What?" Question, or the Gap in Published Studies

Research problems are abundant, yet formulating a researchable problem takes copious reading and razor-sharp precision when crafting the research question. Researchers take great care to make sure the research question arises directly out of the identified problem. A common evaluative question, often used to try to determine the overall impact of a study, is the classic "so what?" question, meant to elicit in a concise manner the most impactful aspect of the designed study. Yet, students often report that this phrase ends up being heard as a declarative condemnation . . . "So what!" . . . mistakenly interpreted to mean that the study has little to no ability to impact overall knowledge and/or impact any practices. Students need to learn that "so what?" questions are designed to help ensure that the needed alignment among the purpose statement, research questions, methodology, and framing of results exists.

When students are asked to deeply consider the potential implications of the research questions they are crafting and to increase the reader's confidence that these research questions are indeed designed to fill a gap in knowledge, they must also be coached to consider whether the new knowledge that may be generated will matter and to whom. That is the ultimate meaning behind the kinds of exercises used to help novice researchers learn to identify and articulate the gaps in the literature that are well-informed, such as illustrated in Exercise 5.6.

Classroom Exercise 5.6. Learning to Locate Researchable Problems

Activities designed to present and reinforce these aspects of designing qualitative inquiry projects can be modified to adapt to various pedagogical contexts.

GOAL: Teach students to learn from published examples, how scholars locate gaps in research and present a logical argument for the purpose of their research.

OUTCOME: Students analyze articles and learn to locate the logical flow of an argument starting with the research problem and ending with the research question.

TIME: 30 minutes

GUIDELINES FOR THE EDUCATOR: Find 3–5 articles based on qualitative studies and bring copies to the class. Organize the class into groups of 4–5 students. Ask each group to take one article and analyze the flow of the article. In addition, ask students to bring a qualitative article to class that is related to their topic. In their groups, give students the following prompts.

GUIDELINES FOR STUDENTS:

1. In your groups, look at the first common article and examine the key phrases the authors use to convey their movement from topic to literature to problem statement to research question. How did the scholars describe how they arrived at the research question? Even if the narrative does not overtly indicate this, can you find the link between these sections?

2. Look at the second article that you brought with you to class related to your own study and do the same exercise given above.

3. Locate the gap as illustrated by the researcher in each article that then leads to the research question.

4. Look at the "Implications" section of both studies and limitations. Are there any gaps that you can find that could lead to further research? Can you think of a research question that you can formulate that leads further from the present study?

5. Is the research significant? What are the areas of contribution—to the discipline and the practice?

These helpful illustrative examples of how scholars discuss an identified gap may serve as models for novice researchers to increase their ability to effectively read published studies as well as increase the likelihood they will craft feasible research questions for their own studies.

Our attempt in this chapter has been to share ideas for teaching a core idea in qualitative research practice—how to find and formulate research problems and craft research questions while keeping in mind the importance and significance of the research itself. Our point in this chapter, is that in teaching students and giving them practice to locate the "gap" in existing research, we also stress the need to help students take this gap and recast it into a researchable question with a clear rationale. In other words, students need to practice how to translate what they find into a research question. We have found the above exercises useful in helping students to craft researchable projects.

CHAPTER SUMMARY ● ● ● ● ● ● ● ● ● ● ●

This chapter sketched out the dimensions of how to approach teaching students about the nature of the research question and how to engage in self-evaluation about the relative strength and weakness of the alignment between the purpose statement and the research question they have crafted. The next chapter tackles ways to think about teaching novice researchers how to construct an effective literature review.

CHAPTER 6

Teaching Students to Write a Review of Literature

A Roadmap, a Conversation, and Metaphorical Imaginations

Writing and synthesizing a review of literature is one of the most daunting tasks for students in research methods courses and yet one of the key skills for graduate success. As mentors of graduate students with a combined experience of working with a large number of committees, we have devised several methods and activities that are helpful to students for crafting a review of literature. In addition, we link the process to the way qualitative analysis is approached so that students see the different applications of qualitative thinking for their scholarly work.

In this chapter, we:

- Discuss how a literature review operates for qualitative inquiry projects and provide ways for faculty to engage students in new ways of thinking about reviewing and applying literature.

- Share a variety of classroom tools, matrices, and activities to approach the teaching of writing a review of literature. These include teaching through metaphors, analogies, stories, and practice prompts.

In Chapter 3, we outlined the different characteristics of holistic pedagogy that apply to qualitative research within critical frameworks. In this chapter, we emphasize two pedagogical approaches—that of inquiry-based teaching and an approach to a flexible and open curriculum. One feature of teaching qualitative research is that it is rarely boring for students. Students conduct field research and studies that keep them enthralled. What could then be easier with regard to teaching qualitative research? One of the main lessons we learned over time is that while students might find the process interesting and entertaining, engagement is another matter altogether. It involves what we stressed in Chapter 4—reflexivity and a constant attention to reflexive processes so that what is read is understood and integrated into the larger picture of what it means to conduct research. It means learning to evaluate, synthesize, and critique readings while giving oneself permission to be bold with writing first drafts.

Teaching the literature review process provides us with several opportunities that can be used for learning and reinforcing these skills and habits of mind. The moments when we are teaching researchers about how, why, and when to conduct literature reviews often contain missed opportunities to further engage novice researchers in the art and science of building questions for critical inquiry (Swaminathan & Mulvihill, 2017) and to further engage them in connecting to the stream of ideas that may impact the project they are shaping. Focusing on pedagogies around teaching novice researchers how to think about a review of literature is also a way faculty can scaffold students to choose between different traditions of qualitative research.

A review of literature is often viewed by students as a behemoth that they have to vanquish, a boulder they have to roll uphill, or a hurdle they have to jump across. A review of literature, as one student put it, "seems to have to do too many things." If faculty who teach students to write reviews of literature reflect on the various objectives reviews have to meet, the task seems onerous. Reviews need to have a narrative, an argument, and reveal a gap to investigate. Rather than gear up for a battle, perhaps a better way to think about the review of literature is to consider it as preparing for a journey or as a way to dialogue and commune with different people and their ideas. Although the term *literature review* suggests a singular type that is self-evident, in reality, there are several types of reviews for different purposes. It is important to clarify for students what those types might be and how to figure out which type of review to use.

The tradition of the review of literature was meant to be exhaustive and exhausting. However, over time, dissertation committees are less interested in seeing evidence of exhaustive (and exhausted students) reviews and are more interested in substantive reviews of literature. This means that rather than read, review, and include every piece of literature associated with the subject, it is more important to choose the seminal works, the works that have had impact, or those that represent a shift in the field or a new development.

What Are the Students' Assumptions of Literature Reviews?

In our courses, we have initiated the conversations around reviews of literature by distributing index cards and asking students to write quick answers to questions regarding their prior assumptions of reviews of literature.

It may be useful for an instructor to do the same by asking students to respond to the following questions:

1. Why should we write a review of literature? or What do you think the purpose is of a review of literature?
2. How do you think reviews should be organized?

Responses to such questions can include:

"It's something we need to do to show the professors that we know the topic well."

"Reviews help us decide what to research further."

"Literature reviews tell me if what I am interested in researching is already out there somewhere."

With regard to organization of literature reviews, the typical responses might range from "chronological arrangement" to "areas that seem to work together."

In all these responses, what novice researchers come into the classroom with is the experience of having completed dozens of final papers for courses where they have often done reviews of literature that have involved examining peer-reviewed articles, looking at what is out there, and trying to put together an argument. It is that memory and socialization that they come into the classroom with, one that then looks at the dissertation process and wonders whether the review of literature is just a mandatory "check-the-box" requirement of the dissertation process. Or as one student complained, "It is supposed to test our endurance."

Communicating to students that the literature review is an argument as much as the problem statement or findings are an argument in the dissertation is a challenge in teaching. Therefore, students need to understand that it is not enough to merely put together a chronological outline of the literature and concepts, although this may be part of what is represented in the review. A thematic review comprising the various ideas and their interconnections that in turn lead up to the argument one wants to make is essential for a literature review to serve the purpose of being one of the main building blocks of the dissertation.

How to Build an Argument in a Review of Literature

To communicate the importance of building an argument that is carefully thought through and is not one-sided, a distinction between an advocate approach and a jury approach is illustrative.

An Advocate Approach

Here the main task of the writer is to present a position and then find evidence to support that position. The term *advocate* emphasizes the intent to communicate a single side of a point of view—an attempt to advocate for one's argument. In this approach, it may be less necessary to consider opposing viewpoints, and is therefore problematic.

A Jury Approach

A jury approach would present arguments in favor of the points one wants to make and also consider critiques of the arguments presented, consider opposing viewpoints, and point out why the view is still worthy, or despite its weaknesses, is still worth considering and in what ways. The jury approach is also the presentation of an argument—yet it is a presentation that includes critiques. Therefore, it reminds students that it is important to critique the theories one builds one's literature around, to critique those arguments and points that one favors or "likes."

In teaching students about literature reviews, one way to address what is traditionally referred to as chapter 2 of a five-chapter dissertation and to move away from a monolithic expectation of a definitive review, is to present the review of literature as comprising varying types. This helps students to realize that there are choices to be made regarding what type of review would fit within the context of their research.

Types of Literature Reviews

There are various approaches to conducting literature reviews and in the next section we provide an overview of some of the most common, and offer a guide to help determine which approach might be best for particular types of qualitative inquiry projects (see Table 6.1). Teaching novice researchers about these processes includes elevating their basic information literacy skills, reinforcing the time close reading requires, and building note-taking frameworks designed to capture the micro and macro levels of comprehension needed in order to craft a sophisticated narration of the selected literature. In addition, each type of literature review holds a slightly different outcome goal and will require a high-level awareness of the specific purpose it aims to achieve in order to not get lost in the weeds.

Descriptions and Discussion:
Thematic, Scoping, and Critical

Thematic Literature Reviews

Thematic literature reviews arrange the literature according to themes rather than chronologically. The researchers need to have a solid command of the literature in order to discern categories of meaning (i.e., themes) from which to organize the selected items. Thematic reviews can be arranged around theories and topics that are relevant to the research questions. The themes ought to tell a story at the meta-level that any single item alone could not tell. Making the case or the argument for why themes are selected is part of the work for this type of review.

TABLE 6.1. Types of Literature Reviews

Type	Central purpose	Function
Thematic review	Organize by theme the central debates of the literature that one is examining.	Explain, justify, and contextualize research questions and methodology in light of the literature review. Thematic organization of the literature can also be used for critical reviews.
Scoping review	To understand and make decisions regarding the scope of the review to determine future research directions. What are the boundaries of the literature that one is going to examine?	Determine future directions of research and questions for research that emerge from the field.
Critical review	Evaluate the strengths and weaknesses of the literature so far.	Like the thematic review, it serves the function of explaining and contextualizing the research question. Critical reviews can contain categories of themes and can overlap with thematic reviews.

Some examples of thematic literature reviews can be found in the following:

Pickles, D., King, L., & Belan, I. (2009). Attitudes of nursing students towards caring for people with HIV/AIDS: Thematic literature review. *Journal of Advanced Nursing, 65*(11), 2262–2273.

Ward, V., House, A., & Hamer, S. (2009). Developing a framework for transferring knowledge into action: A thematic analysis of the literature. *Journal of Health Services Research and Policy, 14*(3), 156–164.

Wong, S., & Sumsion, J. (2013). Integrated early years services: A thematic literature review. *Early Years, 33*(4), 341–353.

Scoping Literature Reviews

A scoping review is undertaken to determine the scope of the literature to review and to place limits on how far back or what types of literature to review. For example, a review of theories can cross disciplines and topics, whereas a review pertaining to a question or issue can be confined to a single discipline or two. Making decisions about which disciplines to include and exclude, and the dates to include and exclude, are all part of a scoping review. Scoping reviews can map the literature to get a snapshot of the range and nature of studies in a particular field. They tend to be more descriptive rather than evaluative in their account. They can also determine whether a systematic review is needed and necessary. If a scoping review determines that not much literature exists in a field or conversely that several comprehensive reviews exist, a decision regarding undertaking systematic reviews can be made. Scoping studies have become increasingly used in order to determine what types of further research is necessary in a given field. Funders of research often commission scoping studies to determine the path of future research.

Examples of scoping reviews can be found in the following:

Connell, J., Barkham, M., Cahill, J., Gilbody, S., & Madill, A. (2006). *A systematic scoping review of the research in higher and further education.* Lutterworth, UK: British Association for Counselling and Psychotherapy.

Cronin de Chavez, A., Backett-Milburn, K., Parry, O., & Platt, S. (2005). Understanding and researching wellbeing: Its usage in different disciplines and potential for health research and health promotion. *Health Education Journal, 64*(1), 70–87.

Davis, K., Drey, N., & Gould, D. (2009). What are scoping studies? A review of the nursing literature. *International Journal of Nursing Studies, 46*(10), 1386–1400.

Critical Literature Reviews

A critical review of literature aims to question and challenge taken-for-granted assumptions and methodologies to investigate a phenomenon. It draws on the literature as a body rather than analyzing individual articles. It also draws on adjacent literature as a creative strategy to stimulate thinking about the content of knowledge as well as the way the research into a particular phenomenon has been carried out. It evaluates the literature for strengths and weaknesses and can help to frame and focus a research project or study. It can also make the researcher alert to themes that may be identified in the study—critical reviews of literature typically tell a story.

Examples of critical reviews of literature can be found in the following:

> Farrington, C. A., Roderick, M., Allensworth, E., Nagaoka, J., Keyes, T. S., Johnson, D. W., et al. (2012). *Teaching adolescents to become learners: The role of noncognitive factors in shaping school performance—a critical literature review*. Chicago: University of Chicago Consortium on Chicago School Research.

> Fu, J. S. (2013). ICT in education: A critical literature review and its implications. *International Journal of Education and Development Using Information and Communication Technology, 9*(1), 112–125.

> Kirkwood, A., & Price, L. (2014). Technology-enhanced learning and teaching in higher education: What is "enhanced" and how do we know? A critical literature review. *Learning, Media and Technology, 39*(1), 6–36.

In addition to knowing and selecting a form of literature review, it is important for novice researchers to name, where appropriate, the specific form of literature review they are undertaking and to make a case for that methodological choice. Making these pronouncements are part of communicating the manner in which some of the most essential ingredients of the project are curated. This level of transparency is not only beneficial for substantiating the design but also for mapping the way the findings may be arranged and discussed.

One of the more important points about reviews of literature is that in terms of a dissertation project, they cannot be stand-alone chapters. Typically, portions of the overall literature review will appear in chapter 1 (introduction/background and problem setting/purpose of the study), chapter 3 (where methodological literature/citations will anchor the methodological thinking and the methods used to carry out the process), and chapter 5 (where a full discussion of the findings in relation to the current state of the literature is crafted). The review will also include the designated chapter 2 (substantial treatment of the literature arranged in a sophisticated manner, guided by the type of literature review deemed most useful to canvas the field, as well as build and shape a persuasive case arguing for the need for the study). While all reviews of literature need a purpose statement and a method attached to them, reviews of literature for a dissertation serve the function of linking the review to the purpose of the study and to the methods.

Scholars may use the terms *conceptual framework, theoretical framework,* or *review of literature* interchangeably, yet there are important distinctions. They all draw on a process of selecting and using literature as evidence for particular claims and set the stage for the kinds of data analysis the researcher has chosen to employ.

Functions of a Literature Review

The purpose of the review is to organize the literature and relevant theories in a way that will showcase the contradictions, overlaps, or adaptations. In addition, the review should point to gaps in the existing research database, and leave room to explain, justify, and contextualize the research questions and methodology that follow from the review of literature. As demonstrated above, there are several types of reviews of literature.

The functions of a review of literature in a dissertation are to:

1. Stand on the shoulders of other scholars—this means to review what came before in terms of the research topic. What questions have been examined? How and what were the results? This examination includes looking at the limitations of existing studies and their strengths so that students can then find a way forward to craft their own research question and defend its significance. This type of review helps to sharpen the research question.

2. Stay mindful of the sense-making processes and find questions that can act as a stimulus for analysis of data.

3. Confirm findings or point out areas where previous research findings may be either presented from a singular perspective or where a better understanding can emerge from new research. A literature review not only showcases the limitations of existing research, it opens up a way forward for new research questions to be asked.

4. Evaluating the existing studies for the types of methods used—checking to see what types of studies have been conducted in the past to be able to "join the conversation" would mean examining the studies to see the methods used. Questions that might serve as checklists for evaluating research articles might include:
   a. What methodology is used?
   b. Is there alignment among the research purpose, the methods, and the findings?
   c. Do the findings answer the research questions?
   d. What are the limitations of the data-gathering methods?
   e. What are the limitations of the study?
5. Tell a story—reviews of literature should make an argument or tell a story through the literature.

Students' Experiences of Crafting Literature Reviews

Students often wonder whether reviews of literature mean only studies are to be cited or should the theories and methods used also be included. The first instinct or first drafts of reviews of literature are often more like annotated bibliographies. Learning to move from summarized lists to making an argument and telling a story is often accomplished through successive drafts of writing a review of literature. Students need assistance with learning how to synthesize and improve the flow of their writing when learning how to integrate the existing literature into their projects. They need practice learning to identify the central concepts and the "big ideas" that are related to their topic of interest.

Tools for Approaching a Literature Review

We developed some tools that we used in our own teaching that have proved to be useful in helping students navigate these confusions. Before we describe these tools, here is a step-by-step list that students may find useful to keep in mind when doing a review of literature.

1. Start with a broad sweep—read some seminal works in the area and some recent literature and look at reference lists to start your reading.
2. As you read, keep track of and decide how far back to go with the literature search. Besides literature from journals and

books, don't forget to look at "gray literature" in the field. Gray literature includes reports from foundations, conference proceedings, and dissertations.

3. Decide what you will include and exclude.

4. Decide what the criteria are for inclusion and exclusion.

5. If there is little literature in your field that addresses your interest, look at a related field for ideas.

6. Use the ideas and charts we have provided in this chapter to keep track of your reading and themes.

7. Study the main arguments or findings from each article.

8. Study the methodology.

9. Compare different articles as you read to see how the same topic has been handled and investigated by different researchers.

10. Think about how it relates to your own research and how it sharpens your perspective and the focus of your research.

Below are a few descriptions of various tools that are useful for keeping track of reading the literature:

- *Concept list, concept maps, and concept art* are ways to build toward synthesis of the selected literature. These tools also help you to make the case for why certain items are included in the review and others are left out. Understanding the limiters and delimiters of the search can be aided by these tools.

- *Checklists* break the tasks into manageable parts to show you incremental progress.

- *Charts* are tools that help navigate the volume and complexity of the resources.

- *Visual diagrams* illustrate the back-and-forth nature of the literature review and show how concepts link together.

- *Tables* can help build a comprehensive database of what literature has been examined and what it contributes to the overall research question. Tables can help students to begin thinking of ways in which to bring the individual articles they read for the review together into themes that will help them synthesize the results or bring the main ideas among several articles together. Putting the research question at the top serves as a reminder to students to keep in mind what they are looking for in an article that will help them in the literature review.

Using Tables in Literature Reviews

In this approach, the articles or authors are on one axis and the main concepts that the student is interested in are represented on the other axis. Taking each article, the student examines whether the main ideas and themes are present and then pulls some relevant quotes to represent the ideas or themes. Such a review would require the student to determine what ideas related to the topic in question are important and then look at whether those ideas are present in different articles (see Table 6.2).

After organizing by article, for a synthesis, the key ideas emerging from Table 6.2 would be used to group themes together. Therefore, it would then lead to a slightly different way of organizing the table or chart. In Table 6.3, the theme is emphasized and different authors discussing the theme are identified.

Table 6.4 can help to organize each article's main points as one reads them and relates them back to the research question that one is investigating.

TABLE 6.2. Organization by Articles and Ideas

Author/article	Idea 1	Idea 2	Idea 3
Name, title, year	Key quote representing idea	Key quote representing idea	Key quote representing idea
Name, title, year	Key quote representing idea	Key quote representing idea	Key quote representing idea

TABLE 6.3. Tools for a Synthesis of a Review of Literature

Research question:

Theme 1 [name the theme]. A theme can be a substantive idea or a review of methods.	Article 1 ideas relating to the theme [cite]	Quotes relating to the theme	
	Article 2 ideas relating to the theme [cite]		How does this relate to the main argument or research question?
	Article 3 ideas relating to the theme [cite]		How do the individual articles relate to one another and to the theme?

TABLE 6.4. Note Taking for a Review of Literature

Citation	Literature review or theories used	Research questions	Methodology	Main findings and interesting quotes	How this fits into your own research question or agenda

Methodological Transparency and Metaphorical Imaginations

Methodological transparency applies to conducting literature reviews as much as it applies to other aspects of research design. Students often need structured assistance to understand why this is essential and then need sequenced ways to practice the related skills. Building literature reviews that are intentional takes time—much more time than what students usually anticipate.

Part of what characterizes the novice researcher is the underestimation of the amount and kind of time needed to read, consider, write, organize written notes, and build usable databases of resources with effective systems for managing references.

Literature reviews are not just scavenger hunts where the energy dissipates when that task is done, but rather they are unique arrangements authored by the researcher to help harness the powerfulness of the existing knowledge on a topic. In Exercise 6.1, novice researchers may be helped by considering various analogies and writing in relation to the review of literature.

Classroom Exercise 6.1. Analogies and Reviews of Literature

GOAL: Stimulate thinking about the review of literature in a variety of ways.

OUTCOME: Students learn to consider reviews of literature as creative ways to think about and situate their research within the context of the work in the field.

TIME: 30 minutes.

GUIDELINES TO SHARE WITH STUDENTS: Share the following list with students and ask them to write a few lines about all the analogies they can connect to reviews of literature.

Are literature reviews more like . . .

1. Writing a shopping list?
2. Conducting a symphony orchestra?
3. Going on a hike along an unknown pathway?
4. Preparing a seven-course meal?
5. Driving a well-known and familiar path from your home to a community park?
6. Visiting an amusement park and trying all the rides?
7. Hosting a dinner party where you can invite only 10 guests (authors of influential literature related to your topic)?

8. Sitting next to a fireplace with a cup of tea and a stack of books and articles to keep you company?

9. Creating a new tune (pattern) from a collection of songs?

10. Creating a collage?

11. Or what combination (or mash-up) of these analogies?

12. Or what other analogy comes to mind for you?

Once students have considered the relative benefits and drawbacks of these various analogies, they can share with their peers and report back to the whole class the analogies that each pair or group found most interesting.

Faculty teaching qualitative research methods can have new starting points for exploring with students the role their starting assumptions about literature reviews play on their planning (or lack of planning) for this aspect of their research project.

Booth, Sutton, and Papaioannou (2016, p. 23) identify four steps for literature reviews:

1. Search.
2. Appraisal.
3. Synthesis.
4. Analysis.

In terms of developing the students' research imagination by which the above steps are accomplished, we refer to Booth et al.'s (2016) four steps as:

1. Being curious.
2. Being discerning.
3. Being contemplative: letting the pieces fall in place.
4. Being critical.

Prepare to Search

We can extend Booth et al.'s (2016) four steps by looking at the preparation needed for a step-by-step search of the literature for relevant articles and books. Reading a general book or article on the topic containing some definitions and citations can be a good place to start. Searching involves systematically keeping notes and lists of names, frequently cited articles, and key terms. These in turn lead to more articles and books.

Searching the literature also means making decisions about the boundaries of the topic. Where will the boundaries of the topic be drawn so that the scope of the search is clear? This includes figuring out what to include and what to exclude so that the focus remains on the research question or the research idea. A key part of searching is also figuring out what to do with the results of the search. It's also important to learn how to file, organize, or collate the different articles into annotated bibliographies in a way that can be useful for summarizing, analyzing, and synthesizing. Searching for articles requires researchers to familiarize themselves with search engines and databases. Boolean searches using the terms *and*, *not,* and *or* can yield different results, as can including terms like *theory* or *definitions* in key-word searches of the topic for review.

Pedagogical Devices for Teaching Novice Researchers about Literature Reviews

Next, we offer some pedagogical devices as tools to help novice qualitative researchers have an authentic experience with constructing an ongoing literature review and what the benefits are of approaching this process as iterative rather than as a singular task to be checked off the project to-do list. Some references to articles and ways of teaching literature reviews that use imaginative methods to discuss how to engage students in reviews of literature follow:

1. Mulvihill's *Moving Into a New Neighborhood* and *Hosting a Dinner Party* analogies (see Mulvihill & Swaminathan, 2017; Mulvihill et al., 2016) resist the "stand-and-deliver" clunky way of writing about the literature.

2. Literature reviews as collage making and roadmap creating—we offer suggestions later in this book about presenting visual displays of data. Those exercises may be adapted for use in literature reviews as well. Students can visually draw or create a collage of similar or contrasting ideas and group them into themes as one of the steps in creating a review of literature. These groups and categories may change and evolve as students come upon new ideas.

3. Small-group literature review teams—students with similar research topics can work together on small teams and share resources. They can also attempt to categorize and write the literature review together.

4. Partnering with reference librarians/information literacy specialists—this is one of the key resources on university campuses that we draw on to help our students.

5. Readers' theater and performing the literature—students can try to perform the literature and have conversations that scholars would have to illustrate the different or similar ideas within the same area of research.

6. Time and task management tools—there are many new tools that students can use for taking notes and for bibliographies and reference list management ranging from Excel spreadsheets to Endnote, Simple Note, or Google Keep. Collaborative writing tools such as Google Docs are also useful for note taking and collaborative writing among student groups.

Critical Reading and Writing: Learning the Vocabulary of Research

When working with graduate students as novice researchers it may often be the case that they vastly underestimate the amount of time it takes to carefully read, take notes, and read again, the materials they have gathered during their search process. They may also need practice learning to carefully review the reference lists of the items they have gathered in order to continue the selection process. Students need to realize the importance of finding the original source rather than relying on a secondary mention of an original source by another author. Most importantly, they need assistance with all aspects of the process of critical reading that leads to critical writing. Breaking this process into component parts and providing scaled-down practice exercises to assist with these aspects of crafting literature reviews may be helpful. Below we provide some additional background and resources to guide those creating and teaching qualitative research methods courses as well as specific exercises that may be useful to use in those courses.

Shon (2015) offers a schematic of codes critical readers can use to learn how to "approach social science journal articles as texts that can be deciphered structurally, mechanically, and grammatically" (p. 3). Shon developed a tool he calls the "Reading Code Organization Sheet" (RCOS) that contains codes he suggests readers use to mark up journal articles. Wallace and Wray (2016) provide a series of helpful suggestions, including reading with purpose. Using your research questions or focused topic area or a *review question* (as termed by Wallace and Wray) to drive your reading will assist with critical reading. As one engages in critical reading, various strategies for note taking can be used. Organizing newly developed questions into categories related to various theoretical perspectives that authors have identified as useful lenses through which the guiding research questions can be viewed is one strategy for organizing the research literature. Various methodological approaches and accompanying methods can be used to access, gather, and analyze data or the key findings of published refereed articles. Most articles are organized first chronologically and then by strength of evidence used to back up the claims, then ranked by overall impact on the way the topic is currently understood. Exercises 6.2 and 6.3 can be useful for introducing students to critical reading while learning the form, structure, and vocabulary of different reviews of literature.

Classroom Exercise 6.2. Analyzing Literature Reviews

GOAL: To teach students how to analyze and unpack literature reviews.

OUTCOME: Students learn to use research vocabulary to write literature reviews.

TIME: 30 minutes.

GUIDELINES FOR THE EDUCATOR: At times, students can accelerate their learning about the form and function of literature reviews by looking for phrases that reveal purpose. Table 6.5 is a short collection of phrases and some corresponding common reasons these phrases are used. Ask students to highlight these phrases in articles or dissertations they are examining and to add to the chart other phrases they believe are useful indicators of purpose.

Exercise 6.3 is an extension of Exercise 6.2 and provides additional practice with deciphering the ways literature reviews are structured.

Classroom Exercise 6.3. Library Excursion

GOAL: Develop a research vocabulary.

OUTCOMES: Students will learn to familiarize themselves with research terms and increase their research and scholarly vocabulary.

TIME: 2 hours.

GUIDELINES TO SHARE WITH STUDENTS: Fill in the Figure 6.1 chart using 10 articles you have located for your literature review.

TABLE 6.5. Examples of Phrases That Can Be Used within Literature Reviews

Phrases	Purpose of the phrase
Conversely, this study or group of studies found . . .	Introducing a set of competing evidence or alternative explanations
The results indicated . . .	A summarization of the results of a single study or a group of studies taken together are suggestive or confirming of a particular finding
Within this sector of the literature . . .	A lead-in to an umbrella statement covering several significant items in the literature
Consistent with previous research . . .	Synthesizing statement about a group of studies or a subgroup of studies in relation to a particular set of findings or claims
Overall, the findings strongly suggest . . .	Synthesizing statement about a single complex study or group of studies

Rubric for Reviews of Literature

Exercise 6.4 can help students create a rubric for the assessment of reviews of literature. This gets students into the mind-set of examining closely what good literature reviews consist of and how to transfer that knowledge into their own writing. Faculty may wish to look at rubrics for reviews of literature such as those provided by Boote and Beile (2005). These may be a good starting point for faculty to share with students in order to help them create rubrics that are targeted to specific reviews of literature—thematic, scoping, or critical.

Classroom Exercise 6.4. How or When to Use Citations and References

GOAL: To remind students of the uses of citations.

OUTCOME: Students learn to be aware of the different times when they need to cite a source.

TIME: 5 minutes plus 5-minute debriefing.

GUIDELINES FOR THE EDUCATOR: As a quick reminder in the beginning or end of a class on teaching students to write the review of literature, here is a 5-minute exercise with a 5-minute debriefing. Although this may seem fairly obvious to many, it is useful to ask students to take an index card and write down two uses for references or citations in their writing of the review of literature. Students can then exchange the cards and share with the whole class any uses that they

Phrase	Full citation of article	Page where phrase is located

FIGURE 6.1. Top ten articles for literature review.

note that are different or ones that they did not think of. Some examples that might come up include (1) acknowledging the source of an idea, inspiration, or a study; (2) pointing the reader to related studies or examples; and (3) acknowledging scholars and writings that have influenced the writer.

This activity encourages students to remain vigilant regarding acknowledging the ideas and writings of scholars in their own work.

CHAPTER SUMMARY ● ● ● ● ● ● ● ● ● ● ● ●

W riting literature reviews need not be an onerous task and can instead be approached in ways that can be imaginative. In this chapter, we offered a variety of ways by which faculty can approach the teaching of literature reviews and offered tools for the organization of the same. In the next chapter, we begin to look at ways to teach the core skills for qualitative researchers that take them into thinking about, trying out, and practicing gathering data.

CHAPTER 7

Participant Observations, Research Questions, and Interview Questions

The Art of Observing and Questioning Self and Others in the Research Process

This chapter explores ways to teach the two mainstays of qualitative research data gathering: participant observation and interviewing. It discusses how faculty can prepare the novice researcher for observing in the field or site and examines the distinction and differentiation between research questions and interview questions. The two are related but not interchangeable—each serves a separate function. Students often confuse the two and/or don't initially understand how to construct either research questions or interview questions. In addition, they underestimate the amount of thinking/writing/revision that is needed in order to produce a refined purpose, research question, and interview questions/prompts.

In this chapter, we:

- Explore teaching the art and craft of interviewing, including determining when it may be appropriate to use a particular type of interview protocol.

- Examine the pros and cons of the various types of interviews: focus and group interviews, narrative and life history interviews, and participatory action research interviewing through collaboration.

- Discuss the ethics related to interviewing vulnerable populations.

The Art and Craft of Observation

Observation is a core skill in qualitative research since observation represents the ability to not only see but to look and take notice. Qualitative researchers utilize observation to read and examine literature, to notice gaps in the existing research, and during data gathering as a tool for data and later analysis to notice nuances, absences, or those subtle points that allow for more layered and meaningful findings. In this chapter, we tackle observations as a data-gathering tool while also pointing out that it is less a mechanical procedure and more an exercise in thinking about what one sees. If the researcher is the instrument of research, as is oft repeated in qualitative research, the observer in qualitative research needs to hone his or her observation skills. Teaching the skill would mean asking students to begin noticing that which they take for granted or observe themselves in relation to their surroundings. While students may already have dipped their feet into such exercises earlier in the semester (see Chapter 3), questions regarding participant observation, what type of observation, and how to prepare to write notes can be addressed in the data-gathering sessions of course work. Although novice researchers often use interviewing as a key data-gathering point rather than observations, social science researchers (see, e.g., Gans, 1999) have pointed out that an advantage to observation is that it allows researchers to see what people do rather than solely relying on what people report they do.

Observation can be a daunting task for researchers who can be confused by what to observe in a site. Too much is going on all the time and it is difficult to make the decision to focus on some rather than other activities. For every decision taken to observe there is a parallel decision that implies one will not observe whatever else might be going on. Novice researchers may either see too many patterns in the field or at the same time wonder whether there are any patterns at all to what they might be observing. Observations in qualitative research are typically participant observations—they are rarely solely observations where the researcher is the complete observer. Participant observation allows researchers to study participants in their environments so that researchers can understand the actions of participants in context and from the perspective of the participants. It helps researchers see what usually occurs on any given day and how participants meet those daily situations.

Although participant observation is a typical norm in qualitative research settings, students are often confused about participation and what it means or entails. Observation appears much more like a real research task or skill—participation appears to muddy the waters. Qualitative research usually involves some type of participation, and the range can span from full participation or even advocacy to minimal participation. Wolcott (1999) uses the term *nonparticipant participant observation* to characterize researchers who while not attempting to hide their role or be covert researchers, nevertheless do not take up the opportunity to participate in the setting any more than absolutely necessary. The question regarding how much or little to participate does not have easy answers. Wolcott further suggests that researchers try to weigh the benefits and losses of different degrees of participation. Each researcher may make a different decision depending on their own personality and comfort zone in a new setting. Some researchers might aspire to be present but forgotten and decide to maintain a low profile, while others might take an active role or might accede to the degree of participation decided on by those in the field.

Powdermaker (1966) suggested that researchers needed to at times be attached and at other times detached, at times "stranger" and at other times "friend." Researchers might, in their zeal to conduct research, forget that they, rather than the participants, are out of place in the participant space. Along the same vein, Gold (1958) outlined four roles that participant observers might play in settings: the complete observer, the observer as participant where the main focus is observation with some participation, the participant as observer where the main focus is participation with minimal observation, and the complete participant. In order to achieve a balance between participation and observation, a balance between involvement and detachment is necessary.

Exercise 7.1 will help students understand the roles and reflect on their effect on the setting and participants. It can introduce students to the varied ways in which one can get involved as a participant in a setting.

Classroom Exercise 7.1. Role Play

GOAL: Students learn what it is like to be a participant observer in a simulated setting.

TIME: 40 minutes.

OUTCOMES: Students learn the skills of observation and learn the multiple ways in which to conduct observational research.

GUIDELINES FOR THE EDUCATOR: Depending on the size of your class, arrange students into groups of five or six members each, with a maximum of six groups. Ask for one observer volunteer from each group to leave the room after giving each observer a sheet of paper that defines his or her role. Inform the observers that they should remain outside or in another breakout room until you send for them. Give each volunteer one of the roles described below, along with brief instructions.

GUIDELINES TO SHARE WITH STUDENTS WHO ARE OBSERVERS: "Each of you has a sheet of paper with role-play instructions. When you are asked to return to class and observe a group, please maintain your role." If there are more or fewer than five groups in the class, these roles can be doubled up or some eliminated. Observers will be invited back into the class once the groups in the class have completed the short reading.

- Observer 1: Maintain no contact with the group. Do not engage with the group. Sit slightly apart or behind and quietly take notes.

- Observer 2: Introduce yourself to the group. Ask the group questions every once in a while. Interrupt them sometimes to talk about yourself and what you are doing there.

- Observer 3: Introduce yourself to the group. Offer to take notes while they talk. Jot down notes and communicate as much as possible non-verbally.

- Observer 4: Introduce yourself to the group and join in as if you were part of the group all along. Ask to read or skim the reading by borrowing it from someone in the group. Jot down notes if you can.

- Observer 5: Play the role of a participant observer using the following principles of good observation: (1) be polite, (2) blend in if possible, (3) do not interrupt, (4) help where you can, (5) find a role you are comfortable with, and (6) write or try to figure out how to write notes as you observe.

The remaining students in the classroom will be given a *short* article on observation or an excerpt from a text they are unfamiliar with to read and discuss. The excerpt could be from any qualitative study that centralizes observations. Classic studies like *A Place on the Corner* (Anderson, 1978/1981) or more recent studies like *Race in the Schoolyard* (Lewis, 2003), *Water in a Dry Land* (Somerville, 2013), or *Consuming Work* (Besen-Cassino, 2014) are examples from which to choose excerpts. Any of these sources can be used to find a short selection for students to discuss observation skills used by the researcher in question.

GUIDELINES TO SHARE WITH STUDENTS PARTICIPATING IN DISCUSSIONS: Read the excerpt silently for 7–10 minutes. Discuss the excerpt in terms of what you can learn about qualitative observations. What strategies did the researcher use that you can infer and what other strategies could have been used?

REFLECTION PROMPTS FOR STUDENTS:

1. What did you think of the "observer" in your group?
2. How did each observer feel about his or her own role in the activity?

Exercise 7.1 is likely to help students become more aware of how they might be seen by participants. In addition, they receive feedback from the groups that have the opportunity to discuss what it was like to have an observer in their midst. By having the observers not read the piece that other students in groups read and discuss, the students playing observer roles are put in the same position as they would be when they enter a site midstream where action is already going on as they arrive and begin their role.

In the reflection discussions, students are likely to talk about their own sense of discomfort at having someone observe them. This helps students understand and empathize with research participants and also brings home the point that it is the researcher who is the outsider in the setting. Observers in turn are also likely to report feeling uncomfortable with the complete observation role or with the interrupting role or the difficulty of finding the right balance between observation and partici-pation. They are also likely to talk about time and the necessity of creat-ing rapport. In addition, they are likely to talk about the many different things they could observe in the short time period and what they focused on. They may bring up what criteria they used to hone in on what to observe or jot down, and what they think they may have missed. They may also discuss the difficulty of taking field notes while observing.

Overall, a role-play activity prepares students for observations in the field—however, role plays are only one way to prepare students for fieldwork. Another way to jump-start discussion regarding roles in the field is to use film. The classic film *The Milagro Beanfield War* (Red-ford & Nichols, 1988) has a researcher from New York University who arrives in New Mexico with a parcel of books and a tape recorder (a point of curiosity for many young students today who cannot recognize what that odd-looking object is). The researcher knows no Spanish and has clearly not prepared himself for his fieldwork in any way, including finding any accommodation for himself. The film clip is a good way to begin a discussion regarding what one can do to prepare for fieldwork even if students are only going to be doing fieldwork locally. Discussions can lead into impression management, learning one's place in a new location, figuring out what to do in a fieldwork setting, and learning the language or the context of research. In addition, it also leads to discus-sions regarding how to gain rapport in the field, identify key players in a context, and identify "gatekeepers" or people at the site who would serve as facilitators for the researcher to obtain in-depth data. Gain-ing trust at sites is crucial for researchers. A second film that is also a good starting point is *Kitchen Stories* (Hamer, 2003). The researcher in *Kitchen Stories* is a complete observer and the silent tug of war for power between the participant and the researcher makes for great dialogue and discussion in class. The film is also a good example of how trust plays a role in researcher–researched relationships.

Helping Students Think through the Focus of Observations

One way to start focusing on what to observe and making decisions is to use the research questions as a guidepost. This allows for adaptation or adjustments to the research questions that may be informed by the observations. Students often face time constraints on their research and data gathering, and lengthy fieldwork times that allow for extended observations in the chosen site are often not possible. In such cases, students usually turn to interview as a method of data gathering, or at times, try to fit in a few sessions of rapid observation. Field observations that are to be fitted into short time frames can be conducted via purposeful observation techniques. It can involve a sheet of paper with some prewritten ideas that can serve as a focus to remind researchers with regard to what they plan to observe.

Wolcott (1999) suggested "ethnographic reconnaissance" (p. 207) as a way to orient oneself in the field. As newcomers to a site, Wolcott's suggestion is to observe without taking notes, and learn about one's site in the way that one might explore a new neighborhood where one has moved in. He suggests a preliminary recording of the observation and writing memos while trying to understand or make sense of what one is seeing in the field. Additionally, he suggests that researchers engage in "ethnographic reconnaissance" periodically in order to obtain an "aerial photo" (p. 214) that can help with the larger perspective of the research and community even while being engaged in a focused role in the field.

In most research books and texts that discuss preparing for the field, it is customary to begin with some short observation exercises. Some faculty like to give assignments to their students to choose a public space, like a coffee shop or a bus stop, and try out observing what is taking place. This exercise can last between 10 and 20 minutes. A few scholars have pointed out that in preparing for fieldwork and observations, great care is taken to ensure that participants are comfortable and attention is paid to the power differential between the researcher and the participants. Reflexivity is brought to the forefront and novice and experienced researchers alike try to ensure that in preparing for fieldwork, they "manage impressions" (Goffman, 1959) and try to blend into their surroundings.

Although most students conduct their observations in places and sites that are relatively safe, some scholars have pointed out that researchers need to take another type of safety into account as well—their own personal safety. Berg (2009) points out that there are two types of risks to fieldworkers: ambient and situational. Ambient risks are risks that are present in the setting and might affect the researcher and the participants equally. For example, an ambient risk in a setting may be the danger of catching a cold or mild infection. Situational risks, however, are defined as those that the presence of the researcher in the setting may bring about. An example of a situational risk is being mistaken for a spy or rival gang member as Venkatesh (2008) was in his study. While there is literature on the risks of fieldwork and how researchers can guard against it by being up-front or being sensitive to fieldwork relations (Loftsdóttir, 2002), much of the literature on the potential for physical harm to fieldworkers glosses over the fact that novice researchers are usually backed by faculty and within institutional contexts where IRBs and personal communications usually prepare the ground ahead of time. However, it is prudent to remind students who are conducting research in new cities, spaces, or groups to be mindful of the setting and to take normal precautions as they would if they moved to a different and new city. Arranging interviews, for example, is best done in neutral spaces rather than in the private homes of participants until one understands the network of field relations better.

Teaching Ideas for Learning to Observe and to Write Field Notes

Learning to write field notes takes practice. Students in class typically tend to write brief notes that are interpretations rather than what they have observed. Bogdan and Biklen (2007), as well as Emerson, Fretz, and Shaw (1995), have discussed how to take field notes and the difficulty of jotting down notes and participating at the same time in the field. Questions regarding what to take notes on, whether one can take notes on casual conversations at a site, or what to summarize and what to elaborate are all typical for novice researchers.

Three main issues need discussion in class: taking notice, writing notes, and recording notes.

1. *Taking notice or becoming aware of (a) surroundings, (b) people, and (c) actions.* For researchers entering the field for the first time, they can try the "aerial view" suggested by Wolcott (1999) and see whether they can draw the site and their specific observation points at the site that might yield the most data with reference to their research questions. A sketch accompanied by notes on what they saw, what they found compelling, and any feelings that the site itself generated are good

first-day notes. In addition, writing what happened, whom they met, and reflecting on their experience is also important.

   2. *Writing or recording notes immediately after the site visit.*

      a. No discussion prior to writing notes. Any discussion regarding "what happened at the site" will inevitably dilute the field notes and is best avoided prior to writing and recording the notes.

      b. Write what happened in any order you remember it and then go back to reorder the information.

   3. *How to record/write field notes.* Field notes will reflect not only what researchers observe in the field but also how researchers observe, what they prioritize, and what networks of relationships they follow or decide to pursue in the context of their research questions. The goal is to "enter into the matrix of meanings of the researched" and experience the events oneself. In the role of researcher, one observes how participants respond to circumstances or challenges or everyday occurrences—writing field notes means taking into account more than only descriptions of what is going on. These descriptions of actions are also interwoven with the researcher's perceptions and interpretations. One way to distinguish between what one sees and what one thinks about what one sees is to ask students to take field notes first by writing what they observed—including dialogue, what people said, and how they acted—as quickly as they can after the event.

   A matrix like the one in Figure 7.1 is an example format for field notes and can help remind students what to include in field notes. Some scholars, like Bogdan and Biklen (2007), suggest a different format with descriptive field notes followed by an observer's comments inserted into the descriptions wherever needed. The notes would follow the format

Date:	Place and time of observation:	Key event/participant pseudonyms:
Field notes: *What happened or what I saw in the field today*	What I think about what I saw: *Here add any questions you might have, musings, issues you might perceive, and interpretations of what you saw or heard*	What I felt in terms of emotions: *Did anything change my thinking? Did I notice anything new or anything that surprised me?*

FIGURE 7.1. What to include in field notes.

where paragraphs of descriptions were followed by consecutive paragraphs of reflection. Not all scholars advise this differentiation. Emerson et al. (1995) warns that dividing the writing of field notes into descriptions and interpretations in the above ways can be misleading. Such distinctions can suggest that descriptions are objective perceptions while interpretations are subjective, when in reality, it is the researcher's gaze, understanding, and unique position that allows the researcher to uncover the particular meaning of an event or action. In this sense, Emerson et al. suggest that findings and method are interwoven and that the discovery of a meaning in the field or from an interview or the sense making that the researcher engages in cannot be separated as subjective acts in opposition or distinctly different and separate from the objective act of seeing. In other words, seeing and perceiving take place simultaneously followed by the reactions of the researcher, and all those together make up field notes.

While we agree with Emerson et al.'s (1995) view that the separation of description and reflection may present a false dichotomy, we also find that in teaching field notes writing, it is easier for novice researchers to learn by separating the two. As researchers gain practice, they can experiment with writing notes and trying different ways to document their thoughts on what they see and experience without sacrificing the "thick description" that comes with narrating their observations.

To help students practice this exercise, we suggest using film clips from documentaries where a lot of action is going on but at the same time, it is easy to explain the context to students. The "Up" documentary series (Almond & Apted, 1964–present) that follows a group of children from the time they were 7 years old and reinterviews them every 7 years is a useful resource for field notes practice. In addition, the film *Miss Evers' Boys* (Sargent, 1997) or excerpts from *High School II* (Wiseman, 1994) can also be used.

In writing field notes, it is possible for different students to focus on different events in the field. They may even describe the same event in different ways, choosing to focus on different aspects of the event. Emerson et al. (1995) give an example of how three people wrote up quite different notes about the checkout line at a grocery store. While one of them focused on spatial awareness, another focused on the relationship between the customer and the employee and other employees portraying the store as a community, while a third described the action in combination with the reactions of the researcher to provide a full account of the researcher's feelings and emotions to the actions and reactions.

Participant observation is a data-gathering method for qualitative researchers—however, it is mediated by the researcher's own gaze and interpretations, since it is the researcher who is the tool of research in the qualitative field. The act of writing field notes has been described by Geertz (1973) as "inscription." According to Geertz, the researcher "inscribes social research, he writes it down. In so doing, he turns it from a passing event, which exists only in its own moment of occurrence, into an account, which exists in its inscription and can be reconsulted" (p. 19). Field notes viewed in this way are more than descriptions—they transform activities taking place in the field into written form. They also represent choices—what the researcher decided was significant and what the researcher decided to leave out. These choices are made in part by what the researcher wants to study but also in part by what the participants find most significant in their contexts and everyday lives. In this sense, inscribing field notes is both an empathetic act as well as one that is adaptable depending on what the researcher might intuit is important to study on any particular day. For example, in one of our fieldwork studies, on one day, without warning, we stumbled upon a group of students who were preparing to teach a class for other students and teachers the following week. Although not in our original plan, which was to study teacher leadership practices, the day and the notes from that day illuminated several aspects of teacher–student relationships at the school and shed light on the ways in which teacher empowerment could facilitate participation in democratic processes on the part of students. Field notes may reflect such decisions that may not have been part of the original data-gathering intent. The lesson for researchers engaged in participant observation is to remain vigilant and attentive in the field. Along with participant observation, interviewing is a core skill for qualitative researchers.

The Art and Craft of Interviewing

Scholars have pointed out that we see interviews everywhere in society—on television, as news, on websites and in newsletters (Patton, 2016), on YouTube, and in other venues. Interview proliferation might lead students to consider interviewing a fairly easy skill to master. However, the opposite is true since interviews can be done well or clumsily, and they can be conducted for different purposes other than social science inquiry. Patton describes several types of interviews and their differing purposes. For example, talk show interviews or celebrity interviews are designed to promote viewership and entertainment while interrogation interviews intimidate or seek a confession, and human resource interviews involve figuring out the fit between the interviewee and the place of employment.

As distinct from the above examples, qualitative interviewing in social science research can be different but equally diverse. Patton (2016) outlines a list of 12 interview approaches: the ethnographic interview, traditional social science research interview, phenomenological interview, social constructionist interview, hermeneutic interview, narrative inquiry interview, life story interview, interpretive interactionism interview, oral history interview, postmodern interview, investigative interview, and the pragmatic interview. The 12 interview approaches range from the completely open-ended interview where the interviewer goes where the participant leads to the completely structured interview where the questions are predetermined and the interviewer strictly adheres to them. While each of these is worth examining for advanced researchers, we have chosen a few general principles of qualitative interviewing to highlight in teaching novice researchers to practice before studying advanced approaches.

We find that teaching question posing and learning the skill of listening and following up with questions are central to learning to be sensitive and skillful interviewers. For this purpose, we use loosely structured interview protocols that allow for changes and adaptations as needed during the course of the interview. Galletta and Cross (2013) regard the semistructured interview as offering various possibilities ranging from open-ended questions to theoretically informed questions. According to Galletta and Cross, semistructured interviews can yield data based on experiences as well as drawn from constructs in the social science disciplines.

In teaching students interviewing techniques, the central task is to teach students to ask the right questions that will elicit conversations and stories, and will privilege participant perspectives. In learning to ask questions, students need to link their research questions to interview questions. As faculty teaching qualitative research methods, we have found that the most important teaching moments occur when students are trying to figure out what their research question is and how they propose to answer the question. Often, students' first instinct is to ask interview questions rather than research questions. In other words, their questions are narrow rather than broad and are probing or follow-up questions rather than an umbrella question that can serve as the focal point of the research purpose. One way to help students to distinguish between research questions and interview questions is to focus on what and how to ask a researchable question. Next, they can learn that a decision on a research question is usually at the end of a series of revisions that are a result of thinking about the research and how to execute it. Chapter 5 offers suggestions to teach students to craft a research problem that in turn leads to a research question.

Alignment among the purpose of the study, the research questions, the chosen methodology, and the selected methods needs constant examination and reexamination in order to determine whether the study's "plumb line" is transparent. Chenail (1997, p. 1) identified the following four parts to a qualitative research plumb line:

1. Area of curiosity.
2. Mission question.
3. Data to be collected.
4. Data analysis procedure.

Patton (2016) discusses the ways in which a research question informs the methods, and the methods in turn reshape and focus the question further. According to Patton, the most important task is to ask questions. The overall research inquiry needs a question or two that can direct the focus of the research. Students tend to describe the phenomenon they wish to investigate in general terms and often forget to move to the second part of the plumb line described by Chenail (1997). The questions themselves need to be open-ended, which typically have the following characteristics: they are not answered with a yes or no, and they are complex questions. Questions are starting points and can evolve over the course of the research. Asking too many research questions in the beginning can result in a lack of focus. While it may be helpful for students to make up a list of questions that they might wish to investigate given the phenomenon of interest, they will also need to focus and direct their questions so that too many lines of inquiry do not emerge. The data to be collected can further help refine the questions. Once the phenomenon is identified and the topic focus is clear, knowing more about where to gather data and who the participants are might help to refocus the questions.

Starting the Conversation: What Are Good Interviews?

Asking students for examples of what they consider good or poor interviews can be a starting point for a discussion in class. Showing clips of talk shows or an interview with a writer and then showing clips from interview studies can help students see what constitutes the interview itself, as well as different types of interviews. Interviewing is an active, dialogic process meant to help elicit deep storytelling in ways that bring forward tacit understandings about the purpose of the study as enlivened by the driving research questions. The interview is a situation where both parties in the dialogue can also construct or represent themselves in particular ways. In this sense, the interview represents a site for identity construction as well as building relationships. Goffman (1959) put it well when he pointed to the mechanisms of impression management in everyday life, a process that all qualitative researchers undertake. To manage impressions is also to present and identify oneself in specific ways that can have an effect on the relationship with the participant. When Nathan (2006) in *My Freshman Year* went to live in the dorms of a college to understand through participant observation the experiences of being a freshman, she wondered how the other students thought of her given the age gap between her and them—she did not fully realize what impression they had of her. The story many of the students had woven had to do with Nathan perhaps being divorced and without money, forced to live in the dorms and go back to school. She learned a great deal from the students while conducting interviews. Interviews allowed her to know more about how students grouped themselves and how they chose their friends, where they met to hang out, and how they made decisions regarding their academic and social lives.

Interview questions are directly related to research questions that in turn emerge from the research purpose. If students can reexamine the diagrams they constructed when thinking of the conceptual frameworks that are foundational to their study (see Chapter 5), they can now proceed to outline the purpose of their research through visual representations and paired writing.

Research questions and interview questions, although often constructed by the researcher in a solo effort, can also be crafted with a peer or in dialogue with an imaginary peer or participant. Research questions lead to interview questions that are in turn openings for dialogue—for the other to speak, share, and open up. They involve conversations, dialogue, and discussions, as well as pauses, silences, and hesitations. They are what Kvale (1996) refers to as "inter-view," where a view is shared between the two people who are conversing. We can go further and say that the interview is also the crafting of a new view in the process of the conversation. It requires the skills of questioning, broaching difficult topics, sensitivity, empathy, and listening. In qualitative interviewing, depth and details matter.

Research Questions and Their Links to Interview Questions

Linking research questions with interview questions is an important step in the data-gathering process. An exercise that reminds novice researchers to connect the two is to ask them to link the interview questions to each research question. A chart that has on one side the research questions and on the other the interview questions can help make the connections clearer. In teaching interviewing skills and crafting interview questions, a classroom exercise that involves interviewing each other can serve as a way to bring up the issues related to interview questions and research questions. Table 7.1 is an example of such a chart or table.

Creating a diagrammatic representation of how all parts of the process—a research topic, a question, a gap, or rationale for the research to occur leading up to a data gathering—go together can help novice researchers keep sight of the big picture. We often post the research question or the main argument of a paper we are writing near our writing desks to remind us of the focus of our work. Similarly, when a project as large as a dissertation is being conducted, it is easy for students to get absorbed in the different aspects so that the big picture gets lost. Continuously working on flowcharts or short diagrammatic representations of the research thus far can work as snapshots of the process that are easy to go back to, trace the developments over time, or make changes and adjustments to the research question and emphasis as the process begins to evolve.

Learning to craft interview questions means thinking about ways to have conversations or dialogue with the participants. Qualitative research designs are flexible to allow for adjustments to take place during the course of data gathering. Qualitative interviews are typically open-ended interviews that have semistructured questions. Preparing interview protocols can take practice and there are different ways to try out interview protocol creation.

TABLE 7.1. Linking Research Questions with Interview Questions

Research question	Interview questions
What are the experiences of first-year teachers in an urban elementary school?	Take me back to your first day here. What was it like? What were some challenges you faced in the first month? • With peers? • With students? • With parents? • With the administration? • With your teaching?
How do urban elementary school teachers explain their teaching philosophy?	Describe what you did in class this week. What led you to choose the activities and learning objectives? What are three things that you find most important for a teacher to do? What beliefs guide your teaching? Can you give an example?

Preparing Interview Protocols: Things to Think About

The rules in qualitative research for preparing to conduct interviews are fairly uniform and advocated by most qualitative research scholars. They are:

1. Prepare to introduce the research topic by letting participants know what is going to take place in the next hour.
2. Begin with a general question about the topic.
3. Begin with a conversational "How are you today?"
4. Begin with plenty of time at hand. (Researchers need to schedule their interviews to leave time before and after for any unexpected events or opportunities that may arise during the course of fieldwork.)
5. Ask questions that are open-ended—avoid questions that can be answered with a *yes* or *no*.
6. Avoid leading questions—questions that lead the participant toward a singular aspect of the issue are leading questions.
7. Ask questions one at a time—wait for the answer to each question before asking the next question.
8. Ask questions that draw out stories—ask for examples or cases or critical incidents rather than seeking out abstract perspectives.
9. Ask questions that seek participant definitions and meanings—be aware of any taken-for-granted vocabulary you might be using as part of your profession.
10. Ask follow-up questions—be ready to veer away from sticking too rigidly to a prepared protocol and go where the story leads.
11. End with the question "Is there anything else you would like to tell me?"
12. End with the question "Is there anything I should have asked you and didn't?"
13. End with the question "Do you have any questions for me?"

Practicing writing interview questions in pairs or in groups of four can help novice researchers look at questions and offer feedback.

While the above checklist can help students craft their questions, Patton (2016), Berg (2009), and Bogdan and Biklen (2007) all offer lists of different types of questions for students to consider. These lists are comprehensive and can be referred to by any novice researcher—however, for the purposes of teaching, we have extrapolated some questions to suggest in class so that students can brainstorm others independently, and in addition, refer to the books suggested. Types of questions for interviews can range from factual to value questions.

Here is a list of the types of questions that we find useful when preparing interview protocols for our projects:

1. Factual questions.
2. Feeling questions (e.g., "How did you feel at that moment?").
3. Perspectives or opinion questions (e.g., "What do you think may be an alternative way to resolve the issue?").
4. Value questions.
5. Critical incident questions (e.g., "Describe a key issue that came up. Describe what stands out in your memory.").
6. Questions that elicit examples (e.g., "Can you give me an example?").

Exercise 7.2 can give students a chance to practice formulating interview questions that relate to research questions.

Classroom Exercise 7.2. Learning to Formulate Interview Questions

GOAL: Practice formulating interview questions from research questions.

TIME: 30 minutes.

OUTCOME: Students learn to formulate interview questions that are related to research questions.

GUIDELINES FOR THE EDUCATOR: Give students some examples of research questions drawn from recent dissertations or from published research studies. Select excerpts—the purpose of the study, the problem statement or rationale for the study, and the research questions—for the students to read. Divide the class into smaller groups of students and have groups try to create interview questions. Prior to starting the *reflection discussion,* distribute the interview questions created by the scholar.

GUIDELINES TO SHARE WITH STUDENTS:

1. Read the purpose statement and the rationale for the study. Read the research question/questions provided by the scholar.
2. Try to come up with a set of interview questions for the participants in

the study. Use what you have already learned in terms of formulating interview questions while constructing this protocol.

REFLECTION PROMPTS FOR STUDENTS: After students have tried their hand at formulating interview questions, share the scholar's interview questions with them.

1. How different or similar are the two sets of questions—yours and those of the scholar?
2. What did you learn from practicing writing interview protocols?
3. Share your questions with your group or with another group in class. Identify and critique your questions and see whether you have asked questions that maintain the arc of a flow and intensity of an interview. In other words, do the interview protocols reflect a beginning, a middle, and an end?
4. Discuss with your peers to see how protocols can be improved.

This activity can help students to examine their interview questions with a critical eye.

Practicing Interviewing with Peers

Trying out research interview protocols with peers or with participants from a similar pool to the research participants are low-risk ways to fine-tune protocols and learn what to adjust in the research questions and interview questions. Scholars (see, e.g., Delyser et al., 2013) have suggested that experiential learning by engaging in peer interviewing and then reflecting on experiences is valuable and can demonstrate to students the richness of qualitative data. Peers can help refine the way in which questions are phrased, clarify that the intent of the interviewer is communicated, ensure that questions can elicit narrative stories by being open-ended, and offer feedback on body language and other nonverbal communicative styles of the interviewer.

Teaching Listening for Developing Interview Skills

Research interviewing comprises dialogue or conversation as well as listening. Holistic approaches to qualitative research emphasize listening as a key skill to be developed among researchers. According to Rinaldi (2006), in *In Dialogue with Reggio Emilia*, listening can be understood as an "interpretive process that does not produce answers but formulates questions" (p. 65).

Listening as a key skill in interviewing has been acknowledged by scholars of qualitative research (Kvale, 1996; Mishler, 1991; Rubin & Rubin, 2011; Seidman, 2005). Jack (1999) offers six different ways of listening in the interview situation. Two of the six ways are used during the process of the interview, whereas the others are more useful during the analysis stages. During the interview, Jack suggests that the researcher engage in "open listening" and in "focused listening." Acknowledging that there is a tension between the two, Jack explains that open listening constitutes paying attention to the emotions during the interview that are experienced by the researcher in response to what he or she is hearing. Body language shifts, tone of voice, and a movement away or toward the researcher are all cues or ways of paying attention to the participant while also engaging in reflexivity regarding the responses in oneself. Focused listening, unlike open listening, is focused solely on the other rather than on the self. In this type of listening, the researcher is searching for commonplace terms that might be used in particular ways by the participant. Jack gives an example of an interview where a woman referred to herself as "dumb." On probing the meaning of "dumb," Jack discovered that to the participant, it did not mean intellectual limitations, but rather a lack of confidence in standing up against people in power. Charmaz (2015) suggests that listening can be analytic. An analytic attitude along with curiosity can lead an interviewer to learn to formulate follow-up questions that are appropriate during the interview process.

In teaching listening as a key interviewing skill, a consideration to keep in mind is the way in which dialogue or the power to speak has been privileged over the power to listen. Students in classrooms who have long been habituated in their schooling to listen rather than speak, may have an understanding of listening as passive or powerless and may not understand the dynamism inherent in the listening attitude. In order to introduce listening as an active skill, we use the brainstorming activity in Exercise 7.3 to discuss what constitutes listening.

Classroom Exercise 7.3. Brainstorming What It Means to Listen

GOAL: To help students think deeply about listening and how their emotions might come into play during the activity.

OUTCOME: Help students prepare for interviewing so that they are aware of the affective dimension of interviews for both the researcher and the participant.

TIME: 20 minutes.

GUIDELINES TO SHARE WITH STUDENTS: Imagine that you have the opportunity to have a conversation and dinner with a person of your choosing. Now, on a sheet of paper, think about the dialogue and your own questions and what might be some answers the person might give. Now think about the ways in which you would listen in such an encounter. Try to fill in the blanks below and use your own metaphors or analogies if you wish.

Listening with . . . (feelings)

Listening to . . . (this could be perspectives, challenging, difficult stories)

Listening for . . . (silences, discomfort, inconsistencies, assurance)

Listening can be . . . (easy, uncomfortable, etc.)

Listening to learn from . . . (participants' perspectives and experiences to add to one's knowledge)

Reflect on the above and give an example of why you think listening might be an active or passive activity.

GUIDELINES FOR THE EDUCATOR: Once students fill out the above on a sheet of paper, have them exchange with two other students and have a small-group discussion. Then have them call out the three most important lessons regarding listening that they shared with one another. Write everything on a whiteboard, take a photograph, and upload to a class discussion board or e-mail to students.

Three points pertaining to listening that can be stressed are the dispositions of *awareness*, *attention*, and *learning* that take place while listening. Further, it is important for students to understand that empathy can lead to discomfort when listening to difficult stories. Students need to be prepared for these feelings and think about how to cope with the impact of stories of displacement, violence, or loss.

Modes of Interviewing: Distance versus Proximity

Interviews are usually conducted face-to-face—however, with the advance in technology and the ready availability of FaceTime, Skype, and Zoom, it is possible to have face-to-face interviews at a distance. Opdenakker (2006) discusses the advantages and disadvantages of interviewing techniques that employ distance or proximity and categorizes interview techniques into synchronous and asynchronous. While face-to-face interviews are synchronous both in time and space, telephone interviews are synchronous in time but not necessarily in space. Opdenakker goes further to categorize e-mail interviews and other Internet modes as also offering possibilities that can be synchronous or asynchronous. In this chapter, we discuss telephone interviews, and in the next chapter, under emergent data collection methods, we discuss the other modes of interviews that utilize virtual spaces.

Phone Interviews

The literature on phone interviews discusses both positive and negative impacts on qualitative data gathering. Critics of telephone interviewing as a data-gathering tool point to the possible detrimental effect on quality and richness of data (Irvine, Drew, & Sainsbury, 2013; Opdenakker, 2006). They point to the difficulty of establishing rapport and lack of visual cues as well as loss of contextual understanding since the researcher would not be able to observe the person in the context of work or place of activity. Other scholars (Mann & Stewart, 2000), however, discuss the possibilities that are presented by telephone interviews including the potential for interviewing participants across larger geographical areas and for interviewing hard-to-reach populations. Some scholars argue that participants may also feel like they have more privacy in phone conversations as opposed to their experiences in face-to-face interviews. In some settings (e.g., hospitals), phone interviews may be preferable because of issues of privacy (see, e.g., Carr & Worth, 2001). Collecting data on sensitive topics via phone may offer the sense of privacy and allow participants to speak more freely. In addition, on the phone, participants have an easier time with interrupting the conversation and ending the interview if they wish to because they do not have to face the interviewer (Saura & Balsas, 2014). Phone interviews require specific preparations that are different from preparing for a face-to-face interview. Here we offer some tips that can be shared with students.

Tips for Phone Interviews

1. Establishing prior contact and rapport. Scholars (Glogowska, Young, & Lockyer, 2011; Smith, 2005) caution against cold calling participants right at the time of the interview and instead go so far as to suggest that researchers establish rapport face-to-face prior to scheduling a phone interview. We suggest that a prior phone call be made where the researcher can perform introductions, clarify the purpose of the interview and the time required, and schedule the interview. This initial call can serve as a way to establish rapport while at the same time checking some functional details like the correct phone number to call. Burke and Miller (2001) suggest setting up interview schedules via phone rather than e-mails, and report that it is valuable to repeat the time and date before ending the conversation.

2. Keeping a record of scheduling processes and a calendar where all the research activities, including the phone interview times, are entered is a useful way to keep all the different data points and calendars organized.

3. Prepare a script and practice with peers to ensure that it is clear, short, and friendly. The description of the study is as important as the tone in which participants are addressed.

4. Think through how to take notes while the interview is being recorded. In phone interviews, taking notes is a less self-conscious activity for the researcher since the participant is not able to view the process.

5. Give a copy of the interview protocol or the topics for the interview to participants so that they get an idea of how the interview will flow. This may allow participants to think about what they might wish to communicate and to explore stories that they might otherwise not remember at the moment of the interview. A note to the participants saying that other questions may follow from the conversation naturally usually helps set the tone of the interview as a dialogue and conversation rather than an interrogation.

6. Test the interview protocol by doing a practice interview.

7. Telephone interviewers need to be mindful of maintaining rapport by starting with informal conversation or general icebreakers.

8. During the interview, researchers cannot rely on nonverbal acknowledgments or support and instead should be prepared to demonstrate responsiveness vocally. Asking for clarifications, statements of validation, or vocalizing support (e.g., saying "uh-huh" or even saying "yes" or "I see" or "I know what you mean") can serve this purpose.

9. Conveying that one is listening in a telephone interview can be challenging. Summarizing and recounting back to the participant can be one way of conveying listening. An example of a summary statement and a follow-up question would be "I am hearing you say that teacher empowerment from the perspective of policy sounds good but that in practice it is complicated. Can you say a little more about how it works in practice?"

10. Drabble, Trocki, Salcedo, Walker, and Korcha (2016) offer the following suggestions and lessons learned with regard to being successful in telephone interviews. Three areas that need to be thought about are (a) maintaining continuous rapport through attention to tone of voice and other positive validatory statements, (b) being responsive and attentive to the participants' views, and (c) ensuring that respect for the

participant and the value of his or her contribution is communicated. We extrapolated the following strategies from participants' suggestions:

a. Being friendly on the phone.
b. Explaining to participants why some questions may sound repetitive, and acknowledging that the previous response was heard and clarifying in what way the current question asked is different from the previous similar one is important so that participants do not feel unheard.
c. Interviewers can hold short conversations that are off-topic as a way to establish continuous rapport. Acknowledging shared experiences with the participants before guiding them back to the interview topics is another strategy for building continuous rapport.

Most of the above suggestions work equally well for face-to-face interviews. However, in-person interviews allow a greater depth of visual cues and nonverbal understanding.

A prepared script to introduce oneself is also important to craft and can be a fun activity for students to practice in class. Asking students to consider and become familiar with some of the following questions ahead of time might help them to think about the interview:

1. What should one include in an introduction to the participant while asking for an interview?
2. Should one talk about the topic of the study?
3. Should one discuss the confidentiality agreement regarding the content of the responses?
4. How should one reconcile the request for asking to record responses while ensuring confidentiality?

Focus Group Discussions and Group Interviews

Like phone interviews, practicing focus group interviews in class can draw from students some typical problems and issues concerning the conducting of focus group interviews. Focus group interviews range from structured or semistructured group interviews to collective discussions or conversations (Kamberelis & Dimitriadis, 2013). Focus groups have usually been used in order to understand the needs of communities, assess resources, or examine the efficacy of a particular implementation. Kamberelis and Dimitriadis outline three aspects of focus groups:

a pedagogical dimension, a political one, and an inquiry-based focus. Within projects that engage in focus group work, any of these dimensions may come into play either singly or in concert with one another. Pedagogically, we can draw upon the relationships between the researcher and the group, examine politically the solidarity or collective action that the group can build, or it can serve as a space where further inquiry can take place. The Freirean pedagogical model (Freire, 1972) is an example of a focus group that has elements of all three dimensions. Focus groups can serve as temporary support groups for participants to feel safe while exploring their lived experiences. Some scholars have advocated homogeneous groups in order to promote community building within focus groups (Madriz, 1997) while others have argued in favor of groups that are diverse (Cammarota & Fine, 2008). For teaching the use of focus groups in qualitative research, the following points are useful to stress.

In focus group interviews, participant selection is often purposeful. It can be based on group membership in a particular activity or at an institution. Focus groups can comprise people from a singular point of view or people with diverse perspectives. Typically, researchers are interested in a diversity of perspectives and yet do not want polarizing perspectives that may lead to conflict within the group. Confidentiality issues in focus groups need to be thought through carefully and articulated within the group. The conversation taking place within the focus group is confidential and participants need to understand that they are trusted to keep it so. Some scholars advise two facilitators for focus groups, with one person moderating the discussion and the other taking notes on nonverbal communications taking place within the group. Some scholars make a distinction between focus group interviews and focus group discussions. The role of the researcher is different in each. In focus group interviews, the emphasis is on group interviews where the researcher takes the lead in asking questions and directing the dialogue. In focus group discussions, the researcher introduces the main topic and perhaps asks a question to start the conversation. The main discussion is left to the participants with the researcher taking a backseat with regard to leading the group. The researcher intervenes only to ask clarifying questions or explanations. Often, the question of how many participants in an ideal focus group comes up. Scholars agree that a focus group needs to be large enough to engage in discussions and at the same time not too large. Usually six to 10 participants make a good focus group with eight being an optimum number.

The following questions can serve as points to ponder when preparing protocols for engaging in focus group interviews or discussions. These points can be distributed to students in class.

Facilitator's Think List

1. Will this be a focus group discussion or a focus group interview?

2. Is the focus group data collection part of other data collection strategies for the research project or is this the sole or primary means of gathering data?

3. What is the focus of the focus group interview? How is the focus related to the research question(s)?

4. What are the multiple roles that the researcher plays in focus group interviews (e.g., this would include facilitator, skillful navigator through any potential conflict, moderator who ensures everyone's voice is heard)?

5. How will issues of confidentiality within the participant group be addressed?

6. Is the group homogeneous or heterogeneous? Is this the most appropriate participant group from which to gather data for the research?

7. Is the moderator/researcher prepared to listen and follow the discussion where it might lead even if the original plan is not strictly adhered to?

8. Is the protocol for the focus group questions open-ended?

9. Is there an additional short questionnaire that needs to be distributed either at the beginning or end to gather any other views that may not be shared in the group?

10. Is it possible to have a co-facilitator to help with observing the group during the sessions?

The protocols for focus group interviews and discussions need to be prepared according to the same principles of other qualitative interviews (i.e., questions need to be open-ended and keep central the research questions).

Narrative Interviews and Life History Interviews

Narrative and life history interviews are also regarded as long interviews in qualitative research. Multiple interviews are usual for life history or narrative interviews. They involve the development of a relationship between the researcher and the participant. They are usually looking to understand the life of the participants in the context of a particular topic or the reverse—looking to understand certain events or parts of their lives in the context of their overall lived experiences. Biographies and autoethnographies, along with life histories, call for longer interviews.

One strategy for long interviews or for narrative interviews is to ask minimal questions that can draw out the life narrative from a participant. The number of questions on an interview protocol may not reflect the time that the interview might take (Berg, 2009). For more on life history interviewing specifics see Mulvihill and Swaminathan (2017).

Recruitment of Participants

Interviewing in qualitative research requires purposeful sampling and recruitment of participants. It is important to think about how to approach participants. At times, if a study is done at an institution or district, the "gatekeepers," or people who can pave the way, need to be identified. Although an initial letter or presentation might be a way to ask for volunteers for a study, nevertheless, it is important to consider how to present oneself and also ensure that participants understand the purpose of the study. In the introduction, there is also the opportunity to share with participants that they are free to decline to answer questions or even stop the interview if they feel so inclined. Although this is emphasized as part of IRB procedures, it serves as a reminder to students that their research participants are volunteers.

Process of Interviewing in Summary
1. Recruitment of participants.
2. Setting up interviews through scheduling time and place.
3. Preparation of interview protocols.
4. Carry with you—interview protocol, IRB consent forms, and questionnaire.
5. Ensure that all technology works and keep a backup.
6. Completion of informed consent and permissions to record.
7. Interview.
8. Post interview—memos and written notes.

The Emotional Work of Interviewing

Interviewing can leave a researcher and participant emotionally affected. Some scholars warn that some participants may regret opening up to researchers and may avoid or act distant the next time they meet the researcher. In addition, listening can affect the emotions of researchers and a gap of a day between scheduling interviews, if possible, would help the recovery of researchers and to assimilate what took place during the interview. Listening to the first interview to think about what might be needed for the second interview is also important preparation for the researcher.

Below are some suggestions to share with students regarding writing memos after interviews.

Postinterview Reflections: Voice Memos as a Way to Reflect on Interviews

Memos can be written, recorded, drawn, or jotted down by researchers. We encourage a wide variety of ways to try out writing memos since memo writing serves as good practice for writing different parts of the research. Although we use the term *record,* we use the term generically to include writing, digital recording, video recording oneself, or jotting down or drawing in a journal.

After an interview, there are thoughts and ideas that bubble up that are outside of field notes. Since most interviews are digitally recorded, it is hard for novice researchers to sit at a computer desk and write these thoughts immediately. In our experience, students generally put those off and as a result by the time they write them, the content of the memos are diluted. Using one's phone can be an easy way to record voice memos on the interview just completed. The memo need not be organized carefully—it is more important to record one's thoughts and impressions. However, three emphases that we would suggest as a quick way to record a memo would be categories of reflecting on the content, the process, and lessons learned.

Reflecting on the Content of the Interview

Regarding content, think about what was intriguing or what was missing that you perhaps expected. A memo regarding what was taken for granted in the interview in terms of content may help the researcher to see what assumptions underlie the stories. Spradley (1987) refers to this process in interviews as "abbreviating" (p. 314), where the participant takes for granted that there is a shared assumption or understanding of a concept.

Reflecting on the Process

Reflecting on the body language of the participant or other nonverbal indications that were noticed by the interviewer should be part of the voice memo. Interview relations between the participant and the researcher can also be recorded here. Were there uncomfortable moments or silences that were awkward? Is it possible to figure out what the participant was willing to discuss and what he or she was unwilling to discuss? Reflecting on the reasons why some topics were not elaborated on could shed light on interview relations or rapport, trust, or perhaps issues of privacy or assumptions regarding shared understandings.

Lessons Learned

What to do for the next time might be useful to record in the voice memo. It also serves as a record for the researcher to take notice of ways to improve on his or her interviewing skills. What could have been done differently can be recorded as well.

Activities for Teaching Interviewing Skills

Exercises 7.4 and 7.5 can be used in conjunction with the content in Chapter 8. Exercise 7.4 is a practice interview in class with two volunteers while the rest of the class observes and offers feedback regarding the interview process.

Classroom Exercise 7.4. The Art and Craft of Interviews

GOAL: To offer students a glimpse of the most common challenges in interviewing.

OUTCOMES: Students role-play interviewing while other students observe the interview and learn the common mistakes made by novice interviewers. Students also learn to give constructive feedback to peers.

TIME: 30 minutes.

GUIDELINES FOR THE EDUCATOR: Ask for two volunteers who agree to role-play interviewer and participant roles. Ask the student playing the participant to leave the room. Brainstorm a broad, general topic and research question that students can relate to for the role play. A general suggestion that usually works is, What does it mean to be a graduate student? Ask the student who is role-playing the participant to return. Have the two students place their chairs in the middle of the room or in the front of the room and role-play. Tell the interviewer that the interview should last between 8 and 10 minutes.

Ask the students who are observing to write down their observations regarding the interview for discussion after the role play.

REFLECTION PROMPTS FOR STUDENTS:

1. What did you think of the interview?
2. What went well?
3. What could have been improved on?
4. What comments do you have about the start of the interview?
5. What can you say about the participant responses?
6. What did you think of the flow of the conversation?
7. How did the interviewer end the interview?
8. What lessons can we learn about interviewing from this role play?

Students' responses to this activity usually bring up the issues that are common to new researchers. They discuss starting the interview, the flow of the questions, and the ending. They also bring up how to read body language and the importance of paying attention to the participant. In addition, they commend the participant role player for sharing his or her views freely. Finally, they discuss the lessons learned from observing the interview.

One of the outcomes of this activity is dependent on the faculty modeling constructive feedback and moderating the flow of dialogue among students so that the lessons learned are meaningful.

Exercise 7.5 allows students some experience of interviewing and gives them the opportunity to try out different modes of interviewing. This activity also takes into account some of the data-gathering practices discussed in Chapter 8 and can be utilized either after the topics in that chapter have been addressed or used as a segue into those topics.

Classroom Exercise 7.5. Interview Modes

GOAL: To experience different interview modes and technology.

OUTCOME: Students experience and learn the promises and challenges of different interview modes that in turn can help them make informed decisions regarding the best way to interview participants for their own research projects.

TIME: 1 hour, including reflection and debriefing.

GUIDELINES FOR THE EDUCATOR: Decide on a general topic for an interview that students can relate to. Divide the class into six groups and give each group one of the following tasks:

Group 1: Interview via phone—prepare a short interview protocol and conduct an interview via phone. In the group, one person will play the role of participant and another the role of interviewer, and others in the group will observe.

Group 2: Interview via Skype.

Group 3: Interview face-to-face and take notes but do not record.

Group 4: Interview face-to-face and record audio on your phone.

Group 5: Interview via e-mail.

Group 6: Focus group interview—one person is designated the focus group facilitator, two to three others as the focus group participants, and at least one observer.

When the groups have completed their brief interviews, they should debrief and reflect on the process.

REFLECTION PROMPTS FOR STUDENTS:

1. What was the experience of conducting the interview?
2. How did the mode of interviewing challenge you?
3. What were some advantages to this mode of interviewing?
4. How can some of the challenges of this mode be overcome?
5. What were the advantages and disadvantages of recording or not recording the interview?

After reflecting within groups, each group can share their experiences with the whole class. This activity allows students to discuss their experiences and learn about the advantages and disadvantages of using different modes and ways of interviewing. They learn how to anticipate and overcome the challenge of situations where recordings may not be possible and learn how to work around technological difficulties.

CHAPTER SUMMARY ● ● ● ● ● ● ● ● ● ● ●

In this chapter, we presented participant observation and interviewing as core methods of data gathering. We offered exercises to facilitate practice in observing, participating, and in conducting interviews, as well as tips for telephone interviews and face-to-face interview preparation. Additionally, preparing interview protocols was discussed. In the next chapter, we continue with data-gathering methods and present activities that can teach students different ways of collecting data besides the participant observation and interview methods.

CHAPTER 8

Teaching Emergent Methods of Data Collection

While much of qualitative research focuses on observations and interviews, the stress is on creating interview structures that are participant oriented. Recent work in qualitative methods that are community, participant, or action research oriented have critiqued the dominantly verbal paradigm of gathering qualitative data and have instead focused on ways to supplement data collection. Data-gathering techniques include the uses of image-based data ranging from drawings and illustrations to photography, photovoice, and video. In addition, data gathering online is explored as a growing area in qualitative research methods.

In this chapter, we:

- Discuss ways that faculty in qualitative research courses can effectively teach these new and emergent methods in data collection.

- Explore issues of participation in gathering visual data and online data.

- Discuss ways to facilitate the teaching of emergent methods.

Teaching Emergent Methods of Data Collection

One of the challenges that faculty teaching qualitative research face is how to introduce students to think about data beyond participant observation and interviewing. Time is a factor in many qualitative research courses and we acknowledge this at the outset. Each of the following modes of data gathering that we outline can be taught as a stand-alone mini-course, perhaps as a 1-credit course that can benefit students who are adept at interviewing and participant observations. However, it is also our contention that these methods can be introduced early, even in an introductory course, so that students can become aware of the multiple forms of data that can be gathered. In our experience, many students find supplemental forms of data that are incorporated into photovoice or videos useful and informative and need to learn about the issues surrounding such forms of data gathering. Multimodal data are in keeping with the multiple facets of qualitative research that can be framed within a holistic pedagogy of qualitative research.

Why Emergent Methods?

Chambers (1997) said that research methods should shift the balance from "closed to open, from individual to group, from verbal to visual, from measuring to comparing" (p. 104). The movement by qualitative researchers over the last few decades to expand the ways in which data can be gathered has opened up the sites that can be explored besides leading to new ways of conducting research. New vistas that can showcase the rich possibilities of qualitative research have opened up to include participants who may be hard to reach; may be in different geographical locations; who may not be physically mobile or be vulnerable for a variety of reasons; and who had previously been excluded from research or whose viewpoints had been marginalized. Teaching qualitative research so that it expands the scope of research participants and spaces is a feature of the holistic pedagogy that we have been sharing in this book thus far. In this chapter, we focus on making meaning from a variety of data-gathering modes, explain their promises and limitations, and offer classroom exercises that help illustrate the critical issues that each can explore.

What Are Multimodal Data?

Data gathering using multiple modes has gained traction in the qualitative research field. Gathering nontextual data has been seen as a response to the overuse of textual data over other forms of communication. While textual or verbal methods demand an immediacy of response from the participants, multimodal data allow participants to reflect and have greater control over the data gathering and production. Twine (2016) critiques the "invisibility of visual culture in research methods," especially in the discipline of sociology (p. 971). Twine's critique of sociology can extend to other social science disciplines and her advocacy of visual literacy as part of research methods courses is important and timely. Multiple forms of data gathering in recent years have included a variety of visual methods, role plays, and panel discussions, as well as walking. While visual methods are not a recent arrival into qualitative research (indeed, photography has a rich history in anthropological field studies; see Bateson & Mead, 1942), photography and other visual- and arts-based methods have come increasingly into use with the intent to decolonize methodology and correct the imbalance of power between the researcher and the participants. Qualitative research practices that go beyond the verbal to the nonverbal and seek to understand the experiences of participants in a variety of ways, are in line with a holistic approach that includes dialogic communication.

One way to get students to think about different methods of gathering data is to first encourage them to see the different phenomena around them that can benefit from qualitative data gathering. Exercise 8.1 encourages students to use their creativity to think about different ways to gather data.

Classroom Exercise 8.1. Brainstorming Interesting Phenomena for Qualitative Research Data Gathering

GOAL: To have students learn to develop awareness and curiosity about phenomena they see all around them.

OUTCOME: Students will learn to ask questions and inquire about the everyday activities they see.

TIME: 20 minutes.

GUIDELINES TO SHARE WITH STUDENTS: Write five types of work or activities of the everyday working life of people that might be interesting to study. Some examples might include a parking meter officer, school crossing guard, or a nail technician. Now, think of five different ways to gather data for each that do not include participant observation or interviewing.

After students have individually thought about the different ideas of qualitative study and data-gathering methods, they can share their ideas in groups of four.

REFLECTION PROMPTS FOR STUDENTS:

1. What were some challenges you encountered with this exercise?
2. What is one lesson you learned from your own thinking, and one lesson you learned after the group discussion and sharing with your peers?

GUIDELINES FOR THE EDUCATOR: Ask students to share the different ways to gather data and ask each group to write a comprehensive list on the whiteboard or on large Post-it sheets.

Ask students to take the different ideas from the Post-it sheets and make one large list for the class to see whether they encompass different ways to gather data. The next activity (Exercise 8.2) is a field activity for students to try out visual data gathering and reflection.

Teaching Visual Literacy

Researchers argue that visual literacy is increasingly important in the world today where technology is at one's fingertips and allows participants and researchers alike to record, create, and produce images of various types. Qualitative research offers us the opportunity to teach visual literacy with a pedagogy of the visual. Visual research demands that researchers be aware of and sensitive to people and places that are photographed. Schratz, Walker, and Wiedel (1995) and Fasoli (2003) regard photographs as having a "power that words often lack" (Wiedel et al., 1995, p. 76). Photographs cannot be regarded as capturing reality nor as depicting the whole truth. Like other image-based data—they are partially constructed by the researcher and the selection and eye of the researcher—circumstances and chance, as well as particular contexts, play a role in what is photographed and what is left out of the picture that is used to tell a story.

Exercise 8.2 introduces students to visual literacy as an important facet to understanding visual data gathering. It is much like the exercises on field observation in earlier chapters. This exercise is designed to get students to think about visual research by considering their own role in decision making regarding what photographs to take, who is the audience, and what are some of the challenges of taking photographs for data collection.

Classroom Exercise 8.2. Keeping a Visual Diary

GOAL: For students to experience using photography or other forms of visual data.

OUTCOMES: Students will learn what it means to use visual data and the advantages and disadvantages of gathering data through images.

TIME: Teaching visual literacy and discussing keeping a visual diary and lesson learned can take up to one full class period of 2–3 hours.

GUIDELINES TO SHARE WITH STUDENTS: Keep a visual diary for 1 week. You may choose any topic that you like or choose an aspect of your life to document.

You could describe through photographs an aspect of your neighborhood or community. Take 10–12 photographs at least. You may do this over the course of several days or use just 1 day for your field diary.

REFLECTION PROMPTS FOR STUDENTS: Write a reflective memo that explains your visual diary and consider the following:

- Discuss what you felt when taking these photographs.
- What decisions did you have to make?
- Did any issues arise?
- What ethical dilemmas, if any, did you face?
- Whose story did you tell with your images?
- Who is your audience?

Points to ponder and discuss in class: Photographs represent a highly selective eye or slice of the truth. In other words, photographs represent "partial truths" (Bogdan & Biklen, 2007) and do not tell the complete story. In addition, it is important to point out to students that photos can be manipulated (Morris, 2011). This exercise can be extended into a class discussion where students can share their visual diaries. In addition, this exercise is suitable for online courses since the visual diary can be uploaded and shared with peers for their comments and discussion.

Below are further issues to consider in image-based data gathering. Some questions to discuss are:

1. What is the researcher's responsibility?

2. How is one to photograph places that might be illustrative of community problems and yet spare the community members embarrassment? For example, Tunnell (2012) asks, How should researchers use a visual qualitative research document or "photograph rural poverty or indications of poverty (e.g., littering) without shaming the people?" (p. 349).

3. How is a researcher to present him- or herself as a participant in the community so that the presence of a camera is not viewed as a threat? Rapport building is as salient to visual qualitative research as it is to interviewing or participant observation. In a surveillance society, as the present is increasingly becoming, a camera can be seen as intrusive and not friendly, an issue that qualitative researchers need to keep in mind while using visual methods. People may wonder, "Why does this person want to photograph me or my store or house?"

Visual qualitative research can be used in empowering and disempowering ways. Students can discuss the ways in which the perspective of the researcher can empower rather than objectify. For example, anthropologists had a history of documenting cultures that they deemed "exotic," and in the process, rendered their participants powerless and distanced them by casting them into objects or the "other." Once visual qualitative research moves from documentation to understanding the world of the participant, the emphasis shifts as does the power.

With the "Keeping a Visual Diary" exercise, students can see what it means to document their experiences or tell the story of a community. They can reflect on the limitations of telling the story from their perspective and what it would add if the community participants could share in the telling of the story.

Multiple Forms of Data Gathering

Multimodal data gathering has allowed for creativity and imaginative possibilities. Several researchers are experimenting with a range of modes of data collection and have reported on the relative success or limitations of their approaches.

In our own search, we came up with the following ways that can be shared with students. While each of these can be explored in depth, a few can be introduced to novice researchers while advanced researchers continue to explore independently.

1. Photovoice (Wang & Burris, 1997).
2. Photo elicitation (Harper, 2002).
3. Video elicitation.
4. Drawing (Kuhn, 2003).
5. Role plays and drama (Guruge et al., 2015).
6. Poetry and writing journals.
7. Walking methodology (Mulvihill & Swaminathan, 2017).
8. Virtual data or online data gathering.

Visual Methods

Visual methods is an umbrella term that comprises a host of different ways to gather verbal and nonverbal data. Putting the power of data gathering in the hands of participants necessitates a research design that is collaborative. Community, action research, or participatory research have all emerged as ways to decenter the researcher and privilege the participant so that participants and the community can own and benefit from the research that they participate in and conduct (Hagey, 1997). Image-based data that are collaborative and directly talk back to research traditions that are tinged with colonial overtones challenge the traditional power relations between the researcher and the participant. They are effective for working with unrepresented populations and hard-to-reach or vulnerable groups, as image-based data are a less intrusive form of research. Moreover, putting data gathering in the hands of participants allows researchers to avoid the "indignity of speaking for others" (Foucault & Deleuze, 1977, p. 209).

Photographs and Visual Data for Empowerment

The popularity of photographs and visual data, regarded as creative methods for qualitative research and interviewing (Rathwell & Armitage, 2016; Wang, 1999), attests to the increasing attention being paid by researchers to multimodal data. Table 8.1 illustrates the ways in which photos are used and the attending terminology.

The ease of taking photographs and uploading them online shifts the relationship that researchers can have with images—moving from thinking of photographs as a means of memorialization to one that communicates. Photographs are tools for communication and community building.

Photovoice Methods for Interviewing

Photovoice has been used in participatory action research and community-based participatory research (Hogan et al., 2014; Wang, 1999; Wang & Burris, 1997). It was developed by Wang, Burris, and Ping (1996) as a way for rural women in China to tell their stories and influence programs that affected them. Photovoice, by putting the camera in the hands of participants, puts power in their hands as they choose how to express themselves and document issues that are important to them. It is an unobtrusive and strategic way to enter the world of the participants, learn what is important to them, and find ways to construct the research problem of interest. Participants in photovoice become coresearchers as they produce and contribute to the data collection and analysis. They take photographs, caption them, and then discuss with the researcher what is going on in the photographs through interviews and focus groups. If we regard vulnerable populations as experts of their own experiences, then dialogue construction is as important as images in visual qualitative research. Woodgate, Zurba, and Tennent (2017) discuss the questions that can guide the follow-up interviews after the photographs are taken. These questions try to get at what the coresearchers see in the photographs, why they think it is taking place, how it relates to their lives, and what can be done about the issue or problem as depicted

TABLE 8.1. Multiple Uses of Photographs in Qualitative Research

Terms	Description	Data collection	Data analysis	Examples
Photo elicitation	The use of photographs as a device or point of reference in interviewing. This involves showing photographs of events or places; the photographs can be researcher or participant generated.	Data may be collected by the researcher or by the participant. Interviews are conducted by the researcher using the photographs as points of reference.	Visual data analysis • Placing photos in social contexts • Understanding why photos were taken (satirize, expose, explain, represent, etc.)	Harper (2002): www.nyu.edu/classes/bkg/methods/harper.pdf
Photo stories	Photos are used as a form of narrative.	Photo diaries, family albums—usually generated by the participant	• Examining photos in isolation versus as part of a group of photos	Brown (2013), Harrison (2002)
Photo collage or photo montage	A blend of images and narrative text where conceptualizing, reflecting, and eliciting are possible.	Photos gathered by the participant and arranged by the participant and/or the researcher. Arrangement by the researcher may reflect several participants' photos to create a montage around a single theme.	• Looking at issues of power: race, gender, power, and sexuality	Gerstenblatt (2013), Vaughan (2005)
Photovoice	Participatory action research method where the participant takes photos to share his or her point of view.	Participant-generated photos	• Examining the significance of the frame of the photo (what was considered significant to photograph)	Wang (1999)
Photo documentaries	Photographs are used to document a life over time. Photo documentary is a term that is often used to document the lives of a group or an individual over the long term.	Photos are taken by the researcher or by the participants. Selection and arrangement is usually done by the researcher.	• Visual analysis combined with interview analysis	Hubbard (2007)

139

in the photographs. Photovoice is anchored in activism and advocacy for vulnerable populations to change conditions for the better.

The goal of photovoice as participatory research is to involve participants in the research process from beginning to end—from the point of crafting research questions and gathering data to analysis and giving their viewpoint in terms of the final write-up. While photovoice has been undoubtedly one of the methods of data gathering that allows participants to have a degree of control over the data gathered, it is also the method that requires that participants be trained in both the methodology and the ethical issues involved. For the safety of the researchers and for the consent of participants, a discussion and dialogue regarding the techniques as well as the social aspect of photovoice needs to be organized.

When teaching qualitative research methods courses incorporating photo data is often an engaging low- or no-cost way to practice data analysis.

Consider trying the following exercise, or some variation of this activity. It is designed to run across two 3-hour class sessions in a workshop mode. Workshop-style teaching incorporates hands-on learning with independent peer learning with the teacher as organizer and facilitator. The workshop style of teaching fits with the holistic pedagogical framework that we advocate throughout this book.

A classroom exercise using workshop pedagogy through which students can try out photovoice research is illustrated below. The instructor should absent him- or herself from the room in order to allow students to build community and negotiate roles. This helps students to identify and grapple with ambiguity—an essential skill for novice researchers.

WORKSHOP: PHENOMENOLOGICAL ETHNOGRAPHY

Using Photos and Other Artifacts to Explore a Cultural Phenomenon

Team up with an interview partner.

PART 1. IN-CLASS PREPARATION FOR NEXT WEEK'S IN-CLASS WORKSHOP

1. 4:00 P.M.–4:30 P.M. Meet with your interview partner to review the instructions for the forthcoming workshop and discuss how you might approach the tasks.

2. 4:30 P.M.–6:10 P.M. Work independently on Electronic Discussion (due next week), which prepares you for the in-class workshop. You are provided with in-class time today *to read and post* so that you can have time to select photos throughout the week.

Below are the instructions you will find on Blackboard for Electronic Discussion.

Read the following materials and create *two original posts* (one related to the readings and a second one that contains your photos) and *two response posts*. Your original posts must include:

1. Original post 1: a reaction to some portion of the readings below.
2. Original post 2: a presentation and an analysis of five to eight photographs that you have taken or found (and included as attachments to your post) that reveal some aspect of the cultural phenomenon (e.g., college or university homecoming) under investigation. These photos are intended to be used for a photo-elicitation conversational interview.

You can perform a Google image search of, for example, "Ball State University (BSU) and homecoming," or explore digital archives of homecoming-related photos, such as the Digital Photo Archives at BSU's Bracken Library, or the *Daily News* photo gallery.

Electronic Discussion Readings

https://files.eric.ed.gov/fulltext/EJ1101721.pdf

http://sweb.cityu.edu.hk/sm6324/Schwartz_VisualEthno_using-photography.pdf

www.qualitative-research.net/index.php/fqs/article/view/1155/2564

www.qualitative-research.net/index.php/fqs/article/view/394/856

http://uir.unisa.ac.za/bitstream/handle/10500/196/ar_schulze_reflexivephotography.pdf?sequence=1

www.jove.com/video/2342/using-visual-narrative-methods-to-achieve-fair-process-clinical

www.ischool.utexas.edu/~yanz/Unstructured_interviews.pdf

http://onlineqda.hud.ac.uk/Intro_QDA/how_what_to_code.php

PART 2. IN-CLASS WORKSHOP, NEXT WEEK

When you arrive in class for Part 2 of the workshop, please have with you a computer, a digital recording device, and a printed copy of your selected five to eight photographs (on regular paper or photo paper) and follow these instructions:

Note: [Insert name of one student] will serve as the timekeeper and taskmaster to help the class adhere to the schedule.

1. 3:30 P.M.–4:00 P.M. Gather in your interview teams to conduct a brief "conversational interview" with each other about the meaning of homecoming as you derived it from *your photographs* and ask each other to recount personal experiences with the phenomenon of "homecoming"

in general, and then personal experiences with a BSU homecoming in particular. This requires you to bring a digital recording device and find a space somewhere in Teachers College to conduct a recordable conversation.

2. 4:00 P.M.–4:30 P.M. Together construct a transcript of the brief conversational interview and post it in this discussion board space.

3. 4:30 P.M.–4:45 P.M. Break.

4. 4:45 P.M.–5:05 P.M. All return to the classroom and then in your interview teams review your transcript and your photos, assign a few codes, and then construct three themes.

5. 5:05 P.M.–5:30 P.M. As a whole class, collectively have a discussion about the phenomenon of homecoming by having each interview team share their photos and their three themes. This will produce a total of 24 themes (8 teams × 3 themes per team). The full class must then decide, out of the 24 themes, how to rework them to arrive at the *five best themes* collectively. [Insert the name of one student] will facilitate this part of the discussion for the class. [Insert the name of two students] will take a series of photos of the discussion with their tablets or smartphones, and then post the photos to this discussion board.

6. 5:30 P.M.–5:40 P.M. Break.

7. 5:40 P.M.–6:10 P.M. *Each person* will create responses to the following prompts and post them in this discussion board space:

    a. Review all of the types of data that were collected and posted in the discussion board and construct an *analytical memo* summarizing your own personal analysis of the phenomenon under investigation. What meaning(s) can be derived from this cultural phenomenon known as homecoming?

    b. Answer the question "What does 'homecoming' mean to you?"

    c. Of all of the photos shared in this exercise, which was your favorite and why?

    d. What was the most memorable moment of today's in-class exercise for you, and why?

8. 6:10 P.M. Done!

When the class returns the next week the faculty member facilitates a debriefing discussion to help draw out the essential elements of what the students learned from this process about data analysis, collaboration, and how cultural phenomena operate within systems of meaning.

The following points can be discussed in class regarding the uses of photovoice and the issues of ethics that arise with using image-based data. Participatory visual research, unlike documentary visual qualitative research, can be empowering to participants and can be a tool for their agency and autonomy. The researcher gives up trying to control the interview encounter and instead empowers participants who can now say what they want and in the way they want.

Performance- and Arts-Based Data

While photovoice and digital storytelling are very popular means of data gathering using visual methods, drawing has also been used by a few researchers as a tool that does not require a digital or technological learning curve. In a study of teenagers' aspirations, Gauntlett (2005) asked the teens to draw celebrities whom they admired and with whom they identified. They were assured that drawing skills were not important. Since the researchers concluded that it would not be possible for them to interpret the drawings correctly, the teenagers were asked to interpret their own drawings through a one-page questionnaire. The teens answered three questions: the first was an open-ended question asking them if they would like to be like the celebrity they chose and the reasons why; the second asked about the choice of the setting in which they drew the celebrity; and the third asked them to choose three words to describe the celebrity which would also be words that they would like ascribed to themselves. The researchers concluded that the drawing process had allowed the teens to develop a more nuanced understanding of the subject matter.

In a study with Kenyan children, Swadener (2005) asked the children to draw before interviews were conducted. The images they drew showed not only their lives as they lived it but also the possibilities they imagined. They drew images of hope and aspiration alongside depictions of everyday strife. Images can be a way for participants to express emotions and feelings, and juxtapose a variety of ideas, actions, and even places and times together. Images can be represented in a nonlinear way and connections that are complex can be made without assigning values or hierarchies to the ideas or concepts. They can instead be represented as equally important within a given context.

Besides visual data, performance-based methods are also increasingly being used to gather data. The use of role plays, drama, and poetry or journal writing may be suggested as ways for participants to express their points of view. In a study with youth, Gillies and Robinson (2012) discuss the inherent difficulties in gathering data from youth with their participation. The first point they make is that youth participation or consent is given on a conditional basis, a point experienced by us in previous research projects (Mulvihill & Swaminathan, 2017; Swaminathan, 1997; Swaminathan & Mulvihill, 2017). A second point raised by Gillies and Robinson is that researchers need to keep in mind that trying to go into schools as adults to gather data from children requires a degree of trust building that takes time. We agree that data gathering with children or youth might not be possible in the short term. Gathering data from populations that are hard to reach requires thinking creatively. It also requires a degree of structure to pursue possibilities. Researchers need to be mindful of other variables that might influence participation—for example, group relations or the mood of the participants or the timing when they are approached for dialogue, role play, or even arts-based data.

Another form of data gathering has been the walking interview or the walking methodology. Used as a pedagogical strategy by Mulvihill (2013) and as a way to mentor students, it is also used as an interview technique by some researchers. Kusenbach (2003), for example, refers to walking with participants while they are engaged in their everyday life as a "go-along" method that might be more conversational and less formal than a structured interview while being less intense than a participant observation setting.

Issues, Ethics, and Best Practices for Image-Based Research

Ethical issues in image-based research can be challenging for researchers. In teaching the practices and uses of visual data, whether from photographs or videos or even drawing, it is important to engage students in a discussion of ethics. For example, how one presents the data collected is a question that needs to be discussed. What types of identifying information is revealed? Do photos reveal particular places? Often, these ethical questions may not be consciously thought through by the participants, making it important for researchers to carefully consider these issues. Marginalized populations might wonder why pseudonyms are needed to protect them, and indeed may also wonder what type of protection they might need at all. Youth, in particular, may resist being "protected," considering it to be synonymous with control by adults. In research using photographs, the following issues need to be considered: (1) Who owns the photographs? (2) Is there informed consent to use the photographs? and (3) Do participants understand the plans for dissemination of the research and of the photographs? Miller-Happell (2006) took photos on loan from participants with the caveat that they would be returned whenever asked for by the participants.

Confidentiality in visual- or image-based research may need to be examined carefully since traditional forms of confidentiality like pseudonyms are inadequate. Instead, informed consent for images needs to be approached with sensitivity so that participants can choose whether to consent to their photographs being used for research purposes and for subsequent publication. In addition to informed consent, the emotional barriers faced by research participants who are taking photographs need to be addressed. If participants are taking photographs of themselves in action, choosing to portray their own communities, or using ways to signify and depict what they want to say with metaphors and different types of images, they may face different challenges than if they were photographing members of the community other than themselves. Hannes and Parylo (2014) conducted a project where they examined the reflections of participants on using photovoice. They found that while some participants enjoyed the photography, others, mindful of the ethical concerns surrounding photographs, tended to avoid using photographs that might be controversial or avoided photographs with people so that they would not have to ask them for consent or have them sign a consent form. Others tended to use photographs that emphasized the background and where people appeared too small to be recognizable, leading Hannes and Parylo to conclude that additional practice might be needed for new participants to start feeling comfortable with asking permission to conduct visual research.

In the next section, we explore data gathering online as an emergent method in qualitative research.

Data Gathering Online

Online research involves two types of research: the first is doing research in the online environment, and the second involves using online platforms such as Skype, Google Hangouts, Zoom, or e-mail. The Internet therefore represents not only a field for research but also a data-gathering instrument. Studies have been conducted in chat rooms, virtual communities, and on social media sites. Analysis has usually been conducted on text already produced on the Internet.

One of the obvious advantages is the low cost of research since participants need not travel, especially over long distances. The ability to use Skype or FaceTime allows for face-to-face encounters, albeit at a distance, so that at least some of the nuances of body language can be observed and questions can be modified according to the nonverbal feedback that one receives. The second advantage of online research is the opportunity and potential for observing social media users—for example, Facebook users or blog participants and authors. Since these activities take place online, cyber research is the appropriate way to examine and understand how participants use these sites. A third advantage of online research is the ability to access hard-to-reach populations. Participants who are geographically separated or are experiencing restricted mobility due to a disability or medication may still be able to meet or be reached via the Internet. One of the disadvantages of online research is that such interviews can also be plagued with technological glitches. Despite increased Internet speed, at times these interviews can be interrupted with some inadvertent "hang-ups." Skype interviews can be rescheduled—however, it may be best to advise students to keep a backup option of a phone interview. Scholars speaking out in favor of video conference interviewing point out that even glitches have their advantages. They argue that the power differential between the researcher and participant can be switched around so that the power to interrupt, reschedule, or even hang up is in the hands of the participants (Saura & Balsas, 2014; Trier-Bieniek, 2012).

Online research often uses preexisting data that are stored and archived on the web. The question that remains less than clear is How is one to use online possibilities for gaining solicited information? Another question that arises frequently is How can participants give informed consent? The Association of Internet Researchers has suggested that researchers need to make it clear that informed consent is required. Kaun (2010), in asking for participation in an online project using online diaries, solved the problem of informed consent on the part of participants by asking people to register and create an account for the online wiki she created for the project. This allowed people to give informed consent as soon as they registered.

Some scholars have pointed out that boundaries between public and private can be more blurred in an online environment but it need not be considered more risky than traditional research (Kaun, 2010; Sudweeks & Simoff, 1999). Researchers cannot be regarded as traditional participant observers in online research. In addition, one of the issues that online researchers face is in integrating online research with off-line data gathering. In an online environment, it may be necessary to gather data both online and off-line so that the two can be blended together in order to be most effective (Sade-Beck, 2004).

In order to teach students how to gather data online and to get an experience of doing so, you can create a blog or wiki for the class. Pinterest can also be used to post images. Students can then partner with each other and practice interviewing online. Allowing students to post anonymously or to create online personas will help them experience the challenges of conducting online research that maintains the pseudonyms or personas adopted by participants while also finding a way to verify that they meet the criteria of purposeful sampling. Turney and Pocknee (2005) used discussion boards in order to conduct online focus groups. As Turney and Pocknee point out, although asynchronicity led to some variations in the type of focus groups that were advocated by Krueger (1988, 1994), they managed to get participants involved in asynchronous discussions and found it to be a superior data collection mechanism for gathering data on attitudes.

Exercise 8.3 gives students practice in gathering data online.

Classroom Exercise 8.3. Data Gathering Online

GOAL: To experience online data gathering and interviewing.

OUTCOME: Students understand the advantages and disadvantages of online data gathering.

TIME: 45 minutes in-class discussion and 1 hour, 30 minutes online. (Data gathering takes place online outside class time. Discussions and debriefing take place in class.)

GUIDELINES FOR THE EDUCATOR: Create a blog for the class. Divide the class into interviewers and participants. Ask the participants to divide themselves into two groups and choose a theme on which they will blog and write a short diary or post photographs, images, or drawings. Ask the interviewers to look at the initial posts and come up with a protocol that has the following components: (1) informed consent, and (2) an introduction and invitation to be a research participant.

Link the blog to the class online platform to allow students to have conversations and interviews. Create groups in the online platform to allow for privacy between group talks. Allow 3 days for the blog posts and 4 days for the interviews to take place. Alternately, allow 1 hour in class time for online interviews.

Have one group of students conduct the interview asynchronously via a discussion board and another group of students conduct the interview via online chat or synchronously.

REFLECTION PROMPTS FOR STUDENTS:

1. What were your experiences of trying out online interviewing?
2. What were some challenges you faced as an interviewer or participant?
3. What were some advantages of this type of interview method?
4. What did you learn about the differences between interviewing face-to-face and online?
5. What ways did you "listen" online?
6. Under what circumstances can we use this method over other methods of data gathering?
7. What ethical issues did you think about when conducting this practice interview?
8. How were emotions conveyed online?

This activity highlights some of the ways in which online interviewing can take place asynchronously and synchronously without visual cues. Students may compare their experiences to those in Exercise 7.4 in Chapter 7, where multiple modes of data gathering (telephone, face-to-face, Skype) were explored. Data confidentiality and richness or depth in data gathering may be topics to discuss after this activity.

CHAPTER SUMMARY ● ● ● ● ● ● ● ● ● ● ● ●

In this chapter, teaching emergent methods of data gathering were explored that make participants coresearchers by engaging them in data gathering. Visual data research methods were described, including photovoice and photo elicitation with classroom exercises for practice and discussion prompts. In addition, conducting online research was also explored. Ethical uses of image-based data and practices were examined with some best-practice suggestions. In the next chapter, we examine creative ways of teaching data analysis.

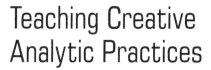

CHAPTER 9

Teaching Creative Analytic Practices

Teaching students how to think about data analysis is a particular type of challenge.

This chapter focuses on:

- Different ways to think about the data analysis process.
- What it means to "analyze data."
- Discussing data management as part of the process of analysis.
- Identifying questions that faculty can use to assist students with scaffolding a more sophisticated and deeper data analysis process.
- Discussing ways faculty can help students ask more effective questions about their data and how this higher-level interrogation impacts their findings and implications.
- Exploring the different ways in which metaphors can be used to facilitate analysis and reflection.

Teaching Creative Analytic Practices

Teaching qualitative research is a rich and exciting experience, one that involves as much learning as teaching. Every text on qualitative research methods explains how to conduct research, and articles based on qualitative research often try to make transparent how researchers undertake the process. However, data analysis in the qualitative research process is often perceived as confusing for both faculty trying to guide students through this process and students trying to heed the advice of faculty not to treat it as a mechanistic or linear activity. There is uncertainty on both sides regarding the lack of a recipe for the work involved. In some respects, qualitative research analysis involves both systematic logical steps as well as flashes of creative insight, intuition, and a process that synthesizes large amounts of patterns in data to produce claims and arguments as results. In this sense, every qualitative researcher, while using all the tools, systems, and steps of analysis and interpretation, also "makes the road by walking"—they each are engaged in their own method-making journey that includes a developmental process of self-awareness. The choices they make influence the types of questions they ask and the analyses of data (Lather, 2006). Teaching qualitative research analysis with such a goal in mind means teaching the structure, scaffolding the reflections, and engaging in discourses to make possible the transformative experiences inherent in data analyses processes, processes that may be different for each student in the class.

Transformative learning theory assists students to change habitual patterns of thinking through a supportive web that includes dialogue, reflection, and centralizing experience (Mezirow, 2003). Teaching data analysis therefore draws from holistic pedagogical principles of transformative learning, where students have to be ready to change their minds, challenge prior assumptions, engage in dialogue and debate with their peers, or be surprised by the connections they make in the data that they had not anticipated. It means creating a classroom space where students have room to experiment and be comfortable with uncertainty. Pedagogical responses to students like "It depends," usually highlight the centrality of context in qualitative data analyses. At the same time, there are some tools that might prompt reflection, analyses, brainstorming, dialogue, and trying out claims based on data.

Data Analysis

Scholars have long raised questions regarding the analysis of qualitative data to produce rich complex analyses and results (Morse, 2004, 2011; Silverman, 2011; Tavory & Timmermans, 2014). Some of the issues with regard to teaching and learning qualitative research begin at the institutional level where due to a single course requirement for qualitative research, teachers of research tend to focus more time on data-gathering strategies rather than analysis (Charmaz, 2015). Scholars have brought up the lack of sufficient numbers of qualitative courses (Benton, Androff, Barr, & Taylor, 2011; Hurworth, 2008) or traced the superficial treatment of qualitative analysis to a general interest in theory or a strong quantitative leaning on the part of students (Raddon, Raby, & Sharpe, 2009). Qualitative analysis has been regarded as difficult to teach (Blank, 2004; Charmaz, 2015; Raddon et al., 2009). Analysis, according to some scholars, is learning to pull apart the data before putting it back together again to tell a story. Pulling apart and putting back together should not be taken to mean that the end result will be similar—a mistake many students make that negates the transformative potential of the data to turn into an argument with evidence.

Scholars offer different suggestions regarding how to approach data analysis with students. Clark and Lang (2002) suggest that trying to teach data analysis along with data collection may prove to be too cumbersome. Instead, they tried to minimize data collection and focus on data analysis by asking students to respond to an image or photograph and used the responses as data and had students write up "field notes" on the responses. Their introduction to data analysis worked well when the image of a person used was not well-known to the students. Charmaz (2015) suggests teaching using grounded theory tools for analysis as a way to build and strengthen the analytical skills of students and move them in the direction of theory construction. She suggests that line-by-line coding can lead to students' starting to theorize about their data in useful ways. Charmaz's coding strategies differ in part from other grounded theory analysts who ask students to restrict themselves to descriptive and thematic initial codes. Instead, Charmaz suggests that students can look for "actions and meanings in short, direct terms and see what happens" (p. 1616).

Blank (2004) points out that while there may be as many as 27 different types of qualitative research (Tesch, 1990), there is nevertheless some degree of unity with regard to data analysis processes. Most data deal with some form of text, and most qualitative researchers, regardless of orientation or adherence to paradigm, are seeking to categorize that text. While these scholars move from data collection to analysis of texts, Miles and Huberman (1994) suggest that data analysis assumes data management, a process that needs to be made transparent to students. They argue that data management and data analysis are linked and cannot be separated from each other. In addition, they explain that data analysis is a series of "concurrent flows of activity" that include data management, reduction, and display.

Teaching Organization: Dealing with Piles and Files

Students usually think that once they have gathered "lots of data" that their job is more or less complete and that the hard part of the research, not to mention the time-consuming part, is behind them. While teaching qualitative research, it is better to unpack what "lots of data" means by reminding students that data collected needs to be substantive, abundant, lush, or thick with examples and stories. However, once students do follow advice and gather the data in abundance, they are confronted with piles and files. Documents and handouts from meetings they attended, audio files from interviews looking deceptively compact in a thumb drive until they are transcribed into 600 odd pages; those field notes they wrote after every interview, the shorthand that looks vaguely familiar that was written after a casual run-in at a grocery store with one of the participants; the phone call that came after the meeting to "explain" what the researcher may have misunderstood; and the list can go on. There are two ways in which students can confront the mountain of data. One is the "drowning in data" syndrome where they are genuinely upset, overwhelmed, and puzzled regarding where to start and wonder whether there is a system or a process that might help them. The second is what we call the "hunt-and-peck" method when students are confident that they know what they are going to focus on. They fast-forward audio files to places where they think they are going to find what they are looking for, a method that is unreliable and leads to overgeneralizations or a polemic-type result where they produce pieces of evidence that support what they think they want to say. Usually this occurs when students are involved with the research to a point where they do not step back from the data to be able to see the whole picture and instead, like the story of the blind men and the elephant, they see only one or two elements and choose to characterize their story from that angle. For students, the completion of data gathering is an emotional moment and one to be celebrated. After celebrations, it is time to turn to data management.

Data Management Plans: Developing Systems to Manage the Data

Novice researchers often underestimate the amount of forethought that researchers need to use as they design qualitative inquiry studies that generally produce copious amounts of data. Systems need to be designed to receive, manipulate, and store data in ways that allow the researcher to have ease of arranging and rearranging the data to create and then test interpretations as they "work the data" toward a coherent narrative of meaning. Data management is organization that forces the researcher to separate and think about the data so that they are sorted into large chunks or categories. The skills novice researchers need to develop in this arena are often sharpened by practice as well as developing the ability to stay flexible and agile as we build the architecture to hold and display the data.

Here are some tools to help novice researchers grapple with various aspects of working with emerging methods of data collection. For example, Penn State Libraries developed a resource to help novice researchers think about data management issues that includes a variety of resources and a toolkit (see *https://libraries.psu.edu/services/research-data-services/data-management*).

In addition, here are a series of prompts for novice researchers to help spur thinking and decision making based on some of the information provided by the Penn State Libraries resources. When creating a data management plan students can benefit from the following considerations:

1. Describing data—build a plan to identify, describe, and label your data.
2. Accessing data—specifically address issues of access and distribution of the data; include in your plan answers to questions such as Who will have access to the raw data? The coded data? The interpreted data?
3. Reusing, archiving, and preserving data—identify and employ a long-term plan for reusing/redistributing, archiving, storing, and preserving data.

Students may also benefit from viewing a TED Talk related to *Rethinking Research Data* delivered by Kristin Briney, a librarian at the University of Wisconsin–Milwaukee (see *www.youtube.com/watch?v=dXKbkpilQME*). Briney (2015) is the author of *Data Management for Researchers: Organize, Maintain and Share Your Data for Research Success* and the blog *Data Ab Initio* (*http://dataabinitio.com*). Asking students to examine these types of resources and to create their own data management plan may help to strengthen many aspects of their research design. To facilitate the process of data management, a sample data management chart (see Table 9.1) might be useful for students to use as a first step to indexing and categorizing their data. To be mindful of time management during the process of data analysis, we added a column that asks students to write down the amount of time they anticipate for each process.

TABLE 9.1. Sample Data Management Chart

Type of data	Needs to be . . .	Status	Questions and reflections	How much time did I spend doing this? What did I learn? (Time management and reflections)
Field notes journal (three in number)	Organized by date and theme, typed or scanned, indexed.	Not done.	Can I just use this as background data and not scan them? Should I categorize by date or site or by person or theme? Or all of the above?	
Audio files	Numbered, pseudonyms assigned for each participant, categorized by date. Transcribed and indexed; I need to go through and add my reflections.	Two sets of interviews are completed out of 16 sets.	Having read the two sets of interviews, I notice that I need to categorize the interviews into themes and people and cross-reference them.	
Photographs	Categorized by participant and by theme; researcher generated and participant generated.	One participant's photos are categorized.	I need to figure out how the photographs relate to the interviews. Did the photographs add to the interview data or vice versa? What did I learn from the photographs?	
Video files	Categorize by participant, date, and theme.	Not yet started.	I need to read body language in the video files as well as transcribe the audio.	
Documents	Categorize by date and theme and determine what documents are needed for analysis and what is needed for background knowledge.	Categorized documents for background knowledge and context.	What do these documents tell me that I do not already know? What documents can be used as historical evidence? What documents can add to the narrative descriptions?	

154

Data Expansion

Although scholars typically discuss data reduction to try to "manage" the piles and files, data expansion is a step that occurs before data reduction. This is the place where the data are sorted out, put into new piles and files, and where one ponders where things should go. We can use the metaphor of organization—the zen of arranging and decor to explain the concept. The idea is to take the large piles of data and see how many different ways they can be sorted initially: by person, date, ideas in each of the datasets, and by new ideas or activities. Imagining, for example, that there is a large garage or store of toys to arrange, asking students to come up with ways to arrange or categorize the toys can be an opening strategy that teaches coding or categorizing. This is the time to brainstorm and think of different ways to categorize or arrange data. Using the toy example, it would mean arranging toys by color, size, activity, age group, skill level, and intent. For example, some toys are geared toward boys or girls, and categories of gender can be thought through and questioned or critiqued.

Data Reduction

The term *data reduction* evokes images of spring cleaning—making one imagine that this is the time to get rid of stuff and keep what is essential. However, this is a term that really should depict focus. Data reduction is a process by which one makes data concise rather than deleting data. Suggestions for data reduction include summarizing interviews through a one-page question-and-answer that depicts what stands out in the data. What topics and issues stand out in this interview? How are they related to the research question? Wolcott (2002) suggests a different way to winnow data. He suggests that researchers take a look at the data and find quotes that seem intriguing or interesting or that spark a question, and put them aside to be used for analysis and interpretation.

Further questions that can be used to help students think about working with data include:

1. How do data analysis procedures vary across qualitative research projects?
2. How do qualitative researchers interrogate data?
3. What are the types of questions one can ask of data and how can one find different ways to think about data?
4. What is the effect of using different lenses to interrogate data?
5. What are the decisions qualitative researchers make when moving from analysis to writing up "findings"?

These questions can be assigned to pairs of students or small groups, as they examine a collection of published studies preselected by the instructor or, if more advanced in their own work, they can examine items they selected for their preliminary literature reviews. The goal is to assist students with developing the critical eye needed to track the data analysis processes used by scholars via their published work. Students also need to learn the vocabulary and language used in data analysis. One way to do that would be to ask students to examine articles and find a list of commonly used terms in the analysis sections of articles to describe what the researcher actually did. Besides building vocabulary, this brings an awareness to students of the variety of ways in which qualitative research analysis can be practiced.

Goals of Analysis

A dialogue or discussion with students on the goals of analysis could serve as an anchor and reminder as to the purpose of coding and creating categories. Students can look at the research questions and determine whether the data collection and subsequent analysis all serve to deepen understanding of the phenomenon in question.

Practical Tips for Handling Data for Coding

There are texts that have been written about coding and the data analysis process (see Saldana, 2015, for a thorough examination of different types of coding)—it is not our intention to repeat what is said in those texts here. Our focus is to suggest the different ways in which teaching data analysis can be explored and the types of teaching assignments or classroom exercises that can facilitate students' understanding of data analysis.

A word about computer coding: there are a number of good programs available for qualitative data analysis that help researchers to categorize and code the text or assign field notes to themes. However, in this chapter, regarding the mechanics of handling data, we focus less on computerized analysis and more on the analytical tools and creative practices that one can draw on to come up with analysis that leads to findings. While students often ask which technique is likely to produce relevant and larger numbers of themes, in our experience, multiple modes of data analysis usually lead to a deeper level of analysis by building on one another.

Data analysis is usually regarded as the "black box" of qualitative research, and scholars, for their part, offer few explanations as to how they moved from coding to interpretation and the telling of the study, thereby inadvertently reinforcing the mystification of the data analysis process.

We offer students the following suggestions when they first begin thinking about handling data for coding and analysis purposes:

1. Read the data several times. Scholars are in agreement that it is important to stay close to the data to be able to analyze them.
2. Cut, sort, and assign codes and themes. Some students prefer to handle data manually and print out the data before cutting and sorting them into multiple files.
3. Keep a list of initial codes and then subsequent lists when you are working on refining codes. Try your hand at different ways to display the data and the relationship between codes and themes.
4. Code several times before you decide you have finished coding.
5. Code and find themes until you can find no new themes in the data or what scholars refer to as the "point of theoretical saturation."

Teaching Students Where Codes and Themes Come From

Codes are usually short terms used as a way to identify action, places, people, or processes in the data. The idea behind codes is to identify similar types of actions or perspectives across datasets, and then try to find nuanced differences among those similarities. For example, how does X think good leadership was exercised in a particular context? And how did Y describe the same incident or context? Did X and Y differ in the ways in which they identified what was "good" about "good leadership"?

Themes are constructs or ideas that can be identified before, during, and after data collection. Themes and codes can come from a variety of places, such as:

1. They can come from the literature—students can comb the literature or use their reviews of literature along with the research questions to come up with codes or themes that they might be interested in pursuing. The danger in doing this is to have preconceived ideas regarding what they want to discover in the data rather than finding in vivo constructs.
2. In vivo codes—in vivo constructs or codes are those that arise from the data alone. They would include "insider" terms, vocabulary used by participants, and participants' ideas and perspectives. The danger in using in vivo codes devoid of examining the

literature is the difficulty in trying to tie the two together after the coding is completed.

3. Codes and themes come from the topic being examined—certain constructs, ideas, and terms get repeated or are particular to a topic or discipline. These need to be considered in coding data.

Giving students a short paragraph from classified ads, Letters to the Editor, or even Yelp reviews or comic strips from a local newspaper would help them see where to look for codes and how they can come up with codes. The following prompts can be shared with students to help them brainstorm themes and codes:

How to Look for Themes or Codes

1. Look at terms that come up repeatedly. What are the words people use repeatedly?

2. Look for terms that are "insider" terms. What are those terms that only those within the group would understand and would need to be explained to a newcomer?

3. Look for typical conversation starters or endings among people if examining focus group data, meetings, or group conversations— they might indicate the type of meeting or conversation. For example, a formal meeting may start in a particular way and may have some rules like minute taking while informal conversations may be more spontaneous or be triggered by questions or practical problems to solve.

4. What is the content of the conversation? What themes do you see being discussed?

5. Look for relationships in the data. Try to find relationships of consistency, relationships that are similar, or those where one is a tool for something else—for example, dialogue is a tool for consensus decision making, or perhaps voting is a tool for the exercise of democratic decision making. Look for relationships that resemble each other or are relationships of function. Each of these would be useful in interrogating the data for themes.

Teaching Analysis as a Collective Classroom Activity

Blank (2004) discusses his experiences with teaching qualitative analysis and concludes that students in his course found generating coding categories and then assigning data to those categories to be most difficult.

Some students tended to procrastinate because they found the task to be overwhelming while others did not schedule enough time for the process, mistakenly thinking that it was a relatively easy task. Blank's experience teaches us that many students consider data gathering to be the most difficult part of qualitative research and that once data are gathered, they imagine that most of their work is completed. One way to help students overcome the feeling that data analysis is too burdensome or overwhelming is to try it in class both in small groups and in a large-group presentation style. Analysis of data or the coding process is still best learned by practice. Students need the classroom space for putting into practice what they learn and to try their hand at the activity several times. For instructors, this means teaching coding and data analysis in class in large- and small-group settings where students can both try it out and receive feedback and guidance. Exercise 9.1 gets students to think about data analysis as a collaborative activity.

Classroom Exercise 9.1. Trying Out Data Analysis in a Large Group

GOAL: Learn to code data in a large group and jump-start the process.

OUTCOMES: Learn how data are coded, how to generate codes, and assign data to codes and vice versa. Learn to analyze and code as a collaborative activity.

TIME: 20 minutes.

GUIDELINES FOR THE EDUCATOR: Select a few pages of interview data from students and display it on a projector. A document reader can do this easily or you can use a word processor to display, highlight, and add notes to text.

Distribute a handout that reminds students that codes can include activity, place, people, interaction, perspectives, or background. In addition, codes can be in vivo or generated from the data and participants' speech or acts, or they can also be theory codes or deductive codes. Begin with in vivo coding as a way to get students to connect with the data. Remind students that you will be showing them partial data and that you will be doing line-by-line coding with the data. Display a page of interview data and ask students to generate codes. Do this collectively as a class with students calling out codes and you typing or writing them down in the margins. A few prompts to students will also generate discussions regarding themes, codes, and the links between each code to generate themes. In addition, ask students whether they can think of how the codes are connected to one another and how each code can be categorized under a theme or subtheme. Ask students to consider how the themes are related to the interview questions and to the research questions of the study. Finally, ask whether students can think of a memo or a claim that they can tentatively put forward given the codes and themes that they have generated so far.

Usually, this exercise energizes students, who then start to think about coding as presenting multiple possibilities, and helps them consider this as an imaginative activity. Students come to realize that research requires one to listen closely to the data in order to synthesize the data, the concepts from the literature, and their own research imagination to then present a claim with the data.

Questions as a Way to Teach Data Analysis

Questions can be used as critical approaches through the entire process of research (see Swaminathan & Mulvihill, 2017, for a fuller treatment of questions in qualitative research). Finding a focus is a recurrent task in data analysis in order to identify and develop key themes to which all individual details of analysis can be related. In order to keep to the focus, different scholars have described ways by which to begin and continue with data analysis that leads to a substantive narrative. For example, Bogdan and Biklen (2007) suggest that data be categorized as settings, definitions, processes, activities, events, and strategies. Each of these can illustrate different action aspects of the data collected. Settings could include the context as well as the physical setting. Definitions would be the category for participants' perceptions and how they define differ-ent concepts or work. An example would be of teachers having different views of what democratic governance meant at a teacher-led school—participants' perceptions regarding objectives would also be classified in this category. Processes would include changes, timelines, procedures, turning points, and transitions. Activities would be regular patterns of behavior and events would be activities that occurred less often of a spe-cific type or nature, and strategies would include friendships, networks, and relationships of various types. While these categories can be one way to organize data, another step that deepens the analysis is to question the data from a variety of perspectives. We outline the five Ws and an H—who, what, where, when, why, and how—to help students move into data analysis by interrogating data after an initial categorization.

Putting the six categories on a sheet of paper and asking students to brainstorm what questions to ask of their data can be followed up with a preliminary list of the who, what, where, when, why, and how ques-tions that we list below. Students can add to these lists and use them to interrogate data. These can be used further in data displays to visually picture which of the participants mention some of the salient concepts or constructs that the researcher finds important to focus on. For example, if examining who mentions race, questions of why, where, and when across participants can lead one to a better understanding of how the data can be analyzed using race as a construct. The same can be done to link gender and work or other identity and activity markers. This type of analytical method is somewhat similar to the constant comparative method advocated by Glaser and Strauss (1967), albeit in a way that allows for a concise bird's-eye view of the data.

Who, What, Where, When, Why, and How?

These questions can serve as a beginning to interrogate data and as a catalyst for thinking in depth. Asking the following questions about each part of the data can help build the analytical structure. Scholars refer to this type of preliminary analysis as open coding or initial coding.

The "Who" Question Can Refer to Any of the Following:
1. Who is speaking here?
2. For whom is this being said?
3. Who is this not referring to?
4. Who is this referring to?

The "What" Questions
1. What is this about?
2. What is the main focus here?
3. What is the process?
4. What is the context?
5. What is the language being spoken (tone, emotion, use of particular words), and what does it connote?
6. What are the consequences of this viewpoint for the purposes of the study?
7. What are the contrasts and similarities in the datasets or in the data?
8. What cultural knowledge is required to read or understand this?
9. What does this remind me of?

The "Where" Questions
1. Where was this taking place?
2. Where in the data does something similar occur?
3. Where in the data does something that contradicts this occur?

The "When" Questions

1. When did the main events or phenomena occur?
2. When (signifying time) did this occur? Draw a timeline to illuminate the main conflicts, agreements, and issues.
3. Why is this occurring at this time?

The "Why" Questions

1. Why is this important or not important?
2. Why does this particular group or person think in this way?
3. Why do people act in this way?
4. Why should we consider gender or race or other identity attributes in analysis?
5. Why did this agreement, conflict, or strategy take place?
6. Why were these decisions made and why were alternatives rejected?
7. Why are some issues voiced while others silenced?

The "How" Questions

1. How does each part of the data relate to the other?
2. How does this contradict other parts of the data?
3. How does this explain questions raised by other data?
4. How does this raise questions about other data?
5. How can I explain or understand the activities that take place on a regular basis in this community?
6. How can I explain or understand the activities that take place suddenly or unpredictably in this community?

Reflective Questions That Interrogate Data

Using reflective questions to interrogate the data can materialize in several ways. For example, there are several good resources to help novice researchers understand a common writing practice called "memoing," which is used to advance the data analysis process on a meta-level, incrementally, as the researcher moves from discrete data units to interpretation to defensible findings. Birks, Chapman, and Francis (2008) provide helpful insights about memoing from the field of nursing studies; Emerson, Fretz, and Shaw (1995) provide an often-used primer on coding and memoing; and Bogdan and Biklen (2007) provide a wealth of pragmatic advice for beginning researchers within education, including tips about memoing and creating observer comments. Each of these resources have high applicability for all types of qualitative inquiry projects.

Using questions to interrogate data can help novice researchers move from one level to the next in data analysis. For example, in one of our classes, a student decided to count how many times a teacher used the word *discipline* in her interviews. While the researcher might learn that discipline indeed was a dominant topic in the interviews, the student would not learn what the teacher meant each time she used the word *discipline* merely through a word count. The teacher might have meant suspensions or calls to the home or referrals. The specific action the teacher was referring to when she used the word would only be illuminated within a context where the data are not merely analyzed as data bits but as part of whole stories.

One of the questions most asked by students is how to assign data to categories. What decisions should one make when assigning data to different categories? Questions that can help students include:

1. Where do I think these data fit naturally?
2. What category or name should I assign the data?
3. How am I defining the category?
4. Are the data an exemplar of the way in which I have defined the category?

Questions for Peer Review

A preliminary analysis of data can be followed up with a class discussion where peers can review one another's systems of analysis. Peer review not only supports the notion of *compagnon*, the French term for a companion on the journey of research, but also teaches one what questions to ask, how to ask the questions, and how to give constructive yet critical feedback. Exercise 9.2 can facilitate students' peer discussions.

Classroom Exercise 9.2. Peer Feedback in Data Analysis

GOAL: Give feedback to a peer by asking questions regarding how he or she analyzed or coded data.

OUTCOMES: Learn to examine how data are analyzed, make connections between analysis and research questions, and learn to give and receive feedback.

TIME: 20 minutes.

GUIDELINES FOR THE EDUCATOR: Ask students to bring one set of field notes or an initial set of codes or categories into which they have organized their data.

GUIDELINES TO SHARE WITH STUDENTS: In pairs, look at each other's initial codes or categories. Share the research question as well as the document that links the research questions to the interview or observation questions or protocols. Looking at the initial set of categories, ask the following questions:

1. What types of things (people, places, activities) did you code/categorize?
2. What other categories might be possible?
3. What categories can be blended or grouped under a larger category?

These initial questions can help students to reflect on the ways they are thinking about the data and open up new ideas.

Once you get the responses from your partner, reflect on the following by writing on an index card:

1. What part of the feedback was easy to hear?
2. What part of the feedback was difficult to hear?
3. How will you change what you have done based on the feedback you received?
4. What did you learn about giving and receiving feedback?

The above activity socializes students to critique and question in constructive ways.

Qualitative Analysis Strategies

Data analysis, as we have mentioned, is best learned by practice. The more a student practices different types of data analysis or tries to see the data in a variety of ways, the easier it will be to stimulate the student into thinking about data in creative ways. Lofland and Lofland (1995) refer to qualitative analysis in terms of strategies that researchers can use. The six strategies they suggest are:

1. Social science framing—Lofland and Lofland suggest looking at data to form an initial hypothesis, argument, or claim.
2. Manage anxiety—they suggest starting analysis early in the data collection cycle; recognizing that data analysis requires more than mechanics; remaining with the task and returning to coding and analysis repeatedly; and finally, using a support group of peers as a way to reduce anxiety.
3. The coding process—the core process of data analysis where the data are broken up or disassembled and categorized.

4. Memoing—the interconnections among ideas, data, and experiences as well as the perspective of the researcher. Scholars have suggested the use of memos as a stepping stone between coding and writing the first draft of the analysis (Bogdan & Biklen, 2007; Charmaz, 2001). Memoing is a way to make sense of the different datasets and sets of codes and themes that serve as a tool for interpretation.

5. Diagramming—Lofland and Lofland suggest outlining a visual display of the relationships between the different codes or themes in the data. Among the varieties of possibilities in data displays, they mention four: concept charts, typologies, taxonomies, and flowcharts.

6. Think flexibly—visual displays can often stimulate flexible thinking as one can try out different arrangements and connections between data as evidence, claims, and concepts.

Teaching Analysis through Visual Displays

Data visualization is a way of data mapping and displaying data. Rom (2015) points out that it is not necessary for a teacher to be an expert on data visualization to be able to facilitate learning it in the research classroom. Admitting to students that we are learning along with them can be a liberating space even if it is an uncertain one. Rom points out that there are two aspects to data visualization: one is aesthetic and the second is technical. Although Rom refers to quantitative data, we think that data visualization activities can be equally applicable to qualitative data. There are several software programs that can be used by students to generate charts, graphs, and scatter plots. Easily available programs like Excel, Word, and Google Charts can all be used for data visualization. In addition, students can use their drawing skills to depict data visually. The intent of data visualizations is to be able to describe the data in a way that is clear and captures the breadth of responses or the different codes or themes. These can be in the form of charts, concept maps, affinity diagrams, tally sheets of themes, or even tables. Shapes and patterns can represent different types of categories. Lines to represent connections between categories can also help depict what data link with what question or what concept. Similar patterns can be highlighted or depicted in one color while contrasts or dissimilarities can be noted in contrasting colors.

There are different ways to visually classify and cross-classify concepts in data. Scholars agree that the classification terms *typologies* and *taxonomies* are most often used synonymously since there is little agreement regarding what differentiates the two (see, e.g., Borgès Da Silva, 2013; Snowden, 2011). Similarly, we do not differentiate between the two and regard both typologies and taxonomies as ways to categorize data and produce what Lofland and Lofland (1995) refer to as an "essential diagrammatic display of all of the forms of the folk or theoretic category being studied" (p. 212) as well as a way to categorize similar actions, places, people, and objects (Berg, 2009). A well-known example of a categorization referred to as taxonomy is Bloom's taxonomy for teaching, learning, and assessment. The progression in Bloom's taxonomy—from knowledge or remembrance to comprehension or understanding, application, analysis, evaluation or synthesis, and create or assemble new work—is an example of how taxonomies can represent different gradations of the same focus area. An example of categorization by typology is the study by Kephart and Berg (2002), who examined 452 photographs of graffiti in a city in Southern California and classified them into five typologies or groups, including publicity graffiti, where the graffiti prominently displayed the name of the gang, and roll-call graffiti, where gang members' names were mentioned. Similarly, they categorized other graffiti according to the content and context or place as threatening graffiti, sympathetic graffiti, and as territorial graffiti. These categories look for nuanced differences and gradations of actions that produce depth and complexity in findings.

Visual displays would try to make connections among these types of parenting strategies. The goal of visualization is to provide an overview of large amounts of data by classifying similar events, actions, objects, people, and places into discrete groups or types.

Concept charts or flowcharts can be made by using software like Prezi that can showcase the different relationships between concepts or demonstrate how an action flows. Many novice researchers like to use large Post-it sheets to draw charts and move them around to rearrange them.

Strauss and Corbin (1990) suggested a tool called a "conditional matrix" by which data can be examined. In this, data are displayed in concentric circles with actions at the center and each concentric circle represents a sphere of influence. Therefore, from the above example of parenting of gifted children, the inner circle might be the action of the child's deliberate practice or hours of study, and the concentric circles would represent influences—for example, one circle could represent parenting support, a second could represent parenting discipline, and a third winning or losing at competitions, and so on. The analysis would start with examining how children react or respond to the different influences on them. Hunter, Lusardi, Zucker, Jacelon, and Chandler (2002) refer to similar visual displays as model making. Making models of data or maps of data in case studies might help students to uncover the complexity of the data and how stories unfold over time. These maps can be made during data collection and again during analysis. Visual learners in particular find data displays or mapping data to be a useful tool for analysis.

Exercise 9.3 can introduce students to constructing data displays. The process involves asking students to take a few sets of data or field notes and then experiment with different types of data analysis methods to produce data displays.

Classroom Exercise 9.3. Creating Visual Displays and Visual Memos

GOAL: Students learn to analyze data through categorization that is visual and learn to regard visual displays as thinking tools.

OUTCOMES: Students create data displays that help them synthesize datasets and assign meanings to categories. They start to make tentative claims about their data.

TIME: 45 minutes, including debriefing and discussions.

GUIDELINES FOR THE EDUCATOR: To create a visual display, students will require substantive sets of data with a focus on the topic or research question. They should bring with them their datasets with initial codes completed. Ask students to read their datasets several times before coming to class. In class, distribute large poster-size Post-its to students or have them use their computers for creating displays.

GUIDELINES TO SHARE WITH STUDENTS: Ensure that you have read the data carefully. The goal is to capture on paper through a visual, the data categories that help you to better understand the datasets. In other words, this visualization is a thinking tool to help you deepen your perception regarding the phenomenon you are investigating. By trying to put data categories and their interconnections in one visual or a series of visual displays, you can start the process of telling a story or making some tentative claims about your data. The following steps will help you go through your data to create the displays. The displays may be regarded as tentative visual memos.

1. Assess materials.
2. Find mutually exclusive categories—this means that data get classified into only one category and not into multiple categories.
3. Place each element into a single category—this means that all the data are exhausted and there are no data that are not coded or classified.
4. Examine these categories and make meaningful connections—this means that there is an attempt to attach some social meaning to the way data have been assigned to categories.

5. Display the data in charts, concept maps, or categories using any graphic organizer that you find useful. Create your own to help make sense of your data.

6. Explain your data display to your peers.

REFLECTION PROMPTS FOR STUDENTS:

1. How did data visualization help you to understand your data in different ways?

2. What tentative claims can you make about your data after going through this exercise?

3. What processes can you explain regarding the content of your data after this exercise?

This exercise helps students to conceptualize their data and think about the data from a different perspective. Students begin to make connections among actions, people, and behaviors while interrogating the data.

Teaching Interpretation

Interpretation is figuring out what the data mean or say about people, groups, or programs that one has been studying. As we have already seen, the process involves taking apart the data, looking at the data, and then reassembling the data to tell a particular story. While some scholars might view this as putting the pieces together like that of a jigsaw puzzle, we think of this as a way by which the pieces come together in a new picture with depth and focus added so that the colors seem brighter or the background clearer. It is more like that of a picture that changes from a two-dimensional image into a moving three-dimensional story. One of the challenges in qualitative data analysis is to ensure that the participants' voices are heard. It is at times easy for researchers to find what they expect, a move that should be resisted. Instead, a reflexive approach toward data interpretation can guard against assumptions and instead allow preexisting ideas to be transformed so that new understandings can emerge. While qualitative research methods are conducive to experiential learning, teaching qualitative methods can use the arts as a strategy for experiential learning (Casey, 2009; Frei, Alvarez, & Alexander, 2010).

Raingruber (2009) assigned poetry to students as a way to initiate qualitative analysis while Lapum and Hume (2015) suggested dance as a way to introduce students to interpretation. Film has also been used successfully as a way to stimulate thinking and analysis. Exercises on interpretation can be useful for practice in the classroom. The deeper meaning of an interaction in qualitative research is possible to glean once one has been in the field long enough to understand "insider" jokes or vocabulary. Nicknames may signify places or events or present a story that led to the nickname. Despite having to become familiar with context in order to begin interpreting observations or interviews, one can practice looking for meaning by interpreting body language in a filmed conversation with the sound turned off.

Faculty can also use the arts, including poetry, film, dance, and choreography to teach interpretation. Interpretation is referred to as qualitative reasoning by Eisner (1997) while meaning making has been likened to magic by several researchers (e.g., Kerr, 1990; Morse, 1994). Teaching interpretation or meaning making through the use of poetry or playwriting involves asking students to take part of the data that they can then perform in class. Performances of data can invoke analytical paths previously not thought about and can centralize action in the data. Writing poetry or converting data into poetry can help students think about distilling meaning. It can also clarify the voices of the participants and distinguish them from the voice of the researcher. Dance is another way to interpret action in the data and tell a story. Art for interpreting data can range from visual displays previously discussed in the chapter to creating storyboards where pieces of the action are depicted through drawings or paintings. Collage can also open doors for analytic thinking. Sommers (1997) used a quilt to represent her own reflections on data. Traditional quilting might seem like a complicated task but can be made easy with the use of paper or Post-it notes that can be stuck on a board or a larger poster paper in different colors and patterns. Like mapping, these are ways that can stimulate divergent thinking so that a deeper analysis is possible.

Use of Metaphor to Teach Qualitative Analysis

Cook and Gordon (2004) explored the use of metaphors to teach qualitative research methods to students studying nursing and suggested that further research was needed on the use of metaphors for pedagogical purposes. Metaphors are powerful means by which people can make sense of shared experiences. Carter and Pitcher (2010) suggested that metaphors are useful to understand similarities and differences between items. According to Lakoff and Johnson (1980), metaphor can be defined as "understanding and experiencing one kind of thing in place of another" (p. 5). They point out that people tend to represent their thoughts or perspectives and behaviors or actions through analogies or metaphors. Metaphors provide an image that suggests a strong likeness to the original idea and communicates meaning.

Life experiences and cultural artifacts are often used as reference points for creating metaphors. In teaching qualitative analysis, we have found the use of metaphors to be particularly exciting for students as a tool to expand thinking about data in different ways.

The use of metaphors in data analysis allows for analysis to be a fun and creative process so that researchers can use imagination and communicate the insights they derive from the data to produce elegant work. In addition, metaphors can be used to get at nuances that may not be overtly evident in the text. For example, emotions conveyed by participants may be better conveyed through the use of a metaphor. Hunter et al. (2002) give the example of trying to communicate the voices of youth resilience. Unlike previous research where resilience is portrayed as the ability to overcome distress without any negative personal impact, resilience research has moved to acknowledge the different ways in which resilience can be experienced and understood. Hunter et al. found that they were unable to capture the myriad ways in which youth responded to resilience until they used the metaphor of a storm and how trees respond to storms. Through the metaphor of storms, they explained the ways in which storms can be sudden, different in intensity and time, and that trees responding to storms could react differently from bending temporarily to growing stronger or to being scarred. Using metaphors allowed the researcher to see the multidimensionality of resilience among youth and to convey its complexity adequately. To teach students how to use metaphor in analysis, they first need to become aware of the frequent use of metaphors in our daily life and talk.

Exercise 9.4 comprises two parts: Part 1 is designed to help students see the metaphors they use in everyday life so that they can identify what are metaphors and analogies. Part 2 is designed to help students learn to analyze data and find patterns and principles from the metaphors used.

Classroom Exercise 9.4. Looking for Metaphors and Analogies

GOAL: Understand how metaphors are used in everyday life and analyze interview data to find metaphors and analogies used by participants.

OUTCOME: Students learn to see their data differently through the use of analogies.

TIME: 40 minutes.

GUIDELINES FOR THE EDUCATOR: Give an example of the metaphors and analogies typically used in qualitative research or in any other activity. We found the following typical terms used by students to describe qualitative research:

Analogies of Travel
- Qualitative research is a journey.
- Qualitative research is a journey of discovery without a map.
- Qualitative research is a maze—there is a pattern but you need to find it.
- Doing qualitative research is like running long distance.

Analogies of Struggle
- Drowning in data.
- Plowing through.
- Wrestling with ideas.
- Juggling too many ideas.

Analogies of Expansion or Learning
- Discovering new things I did not know before.
- Expanding my mind.
- Learning things I did not know before.
- Being surprised by new ideas.
- Being challenged to push my boundaries.

Analogies of Persistence and Athletics
- It's like the loneliness of a long-distance runner.
- The mile 21 block.
- You can make it to the finish line.

After sharing these examples, ask students to complete the exercise given below.

GUIDELINES TO SHARE WITH STUDENTS:

Part 1

Complete any of the following sentences:

- Teaching is like . . .
- Being a [use your own profession here] is like . . .
- Being a doctoral student is like . . .
- The life of a student is like . . .
- Qualitative research is like . . .

After completing the above, share in a small group your writing and thoughts.

Part 2

Take an interview transcript and read it carefully. Try to find the metaphors and analogies used by participants in the interview. What do these metaphors reveal? Are there any patterns to the metaphors or analogies? For example, are they sports metaphors or metaphors of computing? How is work described? What are the comparisons that are made?

Overall, the goal of this activity is to get students to think about their data in depth.

Using Theory as a Building Block for Analysis

Scholars have demonstrated ways to teach analysis through the use of theory. Using theory as a lens through which to conduct analysis is different from using data to build theory. Collier, Moffatt, and Perry (2015) demonstrated three lenses through which the same data can be analyzed. The three perspectives—a sociocultural approach, an ethnomethodological approach, and a rhizomatic approach—all examine and focus on different aspects of the data and the relationship between the researcher and participant. The interview sample was a short dialogue between a child and the researcher. The sociocultural approach focused on the text-making processes of the participant. In that, the researcher examined the data with attention to the actions of the participant and the words or text used by the participant. This case drew on the researcher's own expertise in community literacies. The ethnomethodological approach examined the ways in which both interviewer and interviewee performed during the interview and used technology as a supportive device in the performance. In this instance, it was the participant who requested that he be videotaped, shifting the relationship of researcher and participant in the process. The researcher suggested that if the participant whispered, the researcher would not be able to hear the particpant later on the tape so he in turn suggested that a video might be needed for recording the interaction. A third type of analysis was a rhizomatic approach in which the interaction between the researcher and the participant was analyzed for the affective dimension. The feelings of both, and the place of the feelings within a network of relationships, were the focus of the analysis.

The rhizomatic approach to data analysis (Deleuze & Guattari, 1987), adapted from the concept of how rhizomes grow and evolve, provides an apt metaphor for data analysis processes that defy static codes that often arrive flat rather than three- or four-dimensionally. In addition, this approach to analysis pays attention to nuances that are to do with affect. Theories or methodological approaches can each draw attention to a different focus in the data. In one of our own projects in which we examined and compared video recordings of interviews with transcriptions and texts, we found that a rhizomatic analysis lent depth to our understanding of the affective state of the interviewee and the interviewer, a state not portrayed in the transcriptions. In a similar vein, one of our research projects examined the data from the perspective of three frameworks. The project looked at teacher empowerment and new roles for teachers in schools. Extensive interviews with teachers and with the administration led to many claims. By looking at the data through different lenses, it was possible to make three related arguments with slightly different emphases. The first argument looked at the data through a feminist lens. The argument that could be put forward was one that resonated with teaching being a feminized profession. The extent of empowerment experienced by the teachers could be related to gender and power where the administration was mostly male and the teachers mostly female. A second lens was that of an interpretive lens where an argument could be made of role confusion and misunderstanding on the parts of the administrators and the teachers. If administrators thought they were empowering teachers, teachers on their part did not feel equally empowered and instead thought that empowerment brought status to some and not to others, leading to a hierarchy among teachers where previously there was an equitable power distribution among teachers. A third lens argued that the differences in perception were the direct result of a clash of capitalist values where the teachers represented labor and the administrators represented the owners. The power differential led to a class conflict.

Demonstrating how the same data can be analyzed from different perspectives or lenses can help students think about their data differently. A cautionary note to be aware of in analyzing with a theoretical lens is the danger of fitting data neatly into existing theories. A theory that seems to fit the data completely is both a blessing and a curse. Theory can open up thinking but also limit thought and creativity in analysis. Charmaz (1990) points out that prior theorizing can prevent one from seeing new connections in the data. At the same time, theory avoidance is not the answer either. For novice researchers, it may be important to keep this in mind when analyzing data. The idea behind theory is to find themes in the data that are relevant to the discipline—for example, in social work or education, it may be issues of parenting; in geography, issues of place may be paramount; and in sociology, it may be issues of social conflict.

Research breakthroughs occur when one breaks from one's habitual patterns of thinking so that the same pieces can produce a different pattern. Howard and Brady (2015) outline method as a contested field and the metaphor of research conversations as a way to create a shared vocabulary among students so that students can understand and practice dialogue in ways to advance existing debates. They explain that students can learn the historical contexts of particular methodological innovations through the concept of "contexts of refutation" (p. 523). Understanding what methods were created to refute or challenge existing ways of thinking allows students to see the evolution and context of different methodological developments. For example, feminist methodology was a way to refute the power hierarchies between the researcher and participant.

Jackson and Mazzei (2013) offer some useful ways to think about the complexity of data analysis that may be helpful when you are ready to ease students into the literature advocating for postmethodology. In an introductory course on qualitative inquiry, you might not require students to practice what postmethodologists suggest, but making students aware of the contributions by scholars such as Deleuze and Guattari (1987), Koro-Ljungberg (2016), Lather (2012), Lather and St. Pierre (2013), and St. Pierre (2013, 2015) is important. Here is a short list of some of their work for consideration within course readings:

Deleuze, G., & Guattari, F. (1987). Introduction: Rhizome. In *A thousand plateaus: Capitalism and schizophrenia* (2nd ed., pp. 3–25). Minneapolis: University of Minnesota Press.

Koro-Ljungberg, M. (2016). *Reconceptualizing qualitative research: Methodologies without methodology.* Thousand Oaks, CA: SAGE.

Lather, P. (2012). *Getting lost: Feminist efforts toward a double(d) science.* Albany: State University of New York Press.

Lather, P., & St. Pierre, E. A. (2013). Post-qualitative research. *International Journal of Qualitative Studies in Education, 26*(6), 629–633.

St. Pierre, E. A. (2015). Practices for the "new" in the new empiricisms, the new materialisms, and post qualitative inquiry. In N. K. Denzin & M. D. Giardina (Eds.), *Qualitative inquiry and the politics of research* (pp. 75–95). Walnut Creek, CA: Left Coast Press.

St. Pierre, E. A. (2017). Writing post qualitative inquiry. *Qualitative Inquiry, 37.*

Students in advanced qualitative inquiry courses ought to have a more thorough encounter with these writers while others grapple with the very intriguing epistemological and ontological dilemmas embedded in the activities researchers engage in at all stages of their work.

Some students may find the different ways to analyze data troubling rather than freeing and may try to get from the faculty an answer to the "best way to analyze" data. We have resisted such demands from students by pointing out that analyses begin by exercises that help us to free ourselves to think about the data in a variety of ways.

Writing is part of the analytic and interpretive process as it is part of data collection. Urging students to write before they are ready (Wolcott, 2002) serves the dual purpose of ensuring that students regard writing as continuous and integral to the research process and that it serves as a tool for thinking. Although in qualitative research classes students write continuously, there comes a time when they have to pull the story together and synthesize their data, thoughts, ideas, and the theories they have used to create one coherent narrative.

CHAPTER SUMMARY ● ● ● ● ● ● ● ● ● ● ● ●

In this chapter, we presented different approaches to teaching data analysis. Questions, metaphors, analogies, and theory building, as well as data management and data displays, were described as ways to teach novice researchers how to think divergently about their data. In the next chapter, we look at writing and different ways to approach the teaching of writing.

CHAPTER 10

Writing Qualitative Research Reports and Articles

Writing up a qualitative inquiry project takes a set of special skills, and often faculty find themselves needing to decide how much writing instruction/coaching to incorporate into a course.

In this chapter, we:

- Provide an overview of resources faculty can use to help students learn how to write qualitative inquiry reports and manuscripts for publication.
- Offer explanations regarding what it means to assess qualitative research.
- Offer activities to induct students into a community of scholars.

Assisting students with writing research reports (e.g., course papers, theses, dissertations, conference proposals, refereed journal articles, book chapters) is part of the arc of teaching qualitative inquiry. There are perhaps a few courses at universities that focus totally on teaching qualitative writing, but they are usually for doctoral students (Belcher, 2009, n.d.). Therefore, faculty teaching qualitative courses are usually in the position of teaching everything—conceptualization of a research project, conducting the study, gathering and analyzing data, and the writing up. Understandably, this leaves little time for teaching writing. However, since writing qualitative research is usually built into almost all aspects of the research process, teaching writing is also something to pay attention to all through the teaching process.

In writing qualitative research findings, in particular, scholars have pointed out that the better qualitative studies often read like stories—they are compelling, persuasive, and evocative—as opposed to those that read like manuals or a dry report of events. The studies that tell a compelling story are usually those that also incorporate an insight and are nuanced and multilayered. They have also been well marinated by the researcher's thinking and have been subject to repeated kneading like one does with a bowl of flour and water to bake an elegant loaf of bread. The final work involves creativity (Morse, 1994; Mulvihill & Swaminathan, 2012a, 2012b, 2013) and a spirit of exploration and adventure. However, in the pedagogical realm, it is not entirely clear how, as faculty, we can teach qualitative research and possibly communicate this rather indescribable process to students and have them understand and then try it out.

Some early effective advice-giving books related to these pedagogical acts include Becker's (2010) *Writing for Social Scientists: How to Start and Finish Your Thesis, Book, or Article*; Van Maanen's (2011) *Tales of the Field: On Writing Ethnography*; and Wolcott's (2001) *Writing Up Qualitative Research*. Many have benefited from Bogdan and Biklen's (2007) "Writing It Up" chapter in their *Qualitative Research for Education,* as well as Richardson and St. Pierre's (2005) chapter "Writing: A Method of Inquiry," in *The Sage Handbook of Qualitative Research.* Most recently, scholars are reading Sword's two books, *Stylish Academic Writing* (2012) and *Air and Light and Time and Space: How Successful Academics Write* (2017), as well as Singh and Lukkarila's (2017) *Successful Academic Writing: A Complete Guide for Social and Behavioral Scientists,* a highly engaging and practical text. And finally, many continue to use Zinsser's (1983, 2012) highly celebrated *On Writing Well.*

Teaching novice qualitative researchers how to prepare research reports and learn how to fashion manuscripts for publication is predicated on the degree to which they have already developed an identity as a writer; most students report they have not intentionally worked to create this aspect of their identity. Learning to be a successful writer is a dimension that can occupy one objective of qualitative research methods courses and there are very interesting and helpful resources that exist to help bring this aspect of the course design to life. For example, Huff summarizes her insights into what it takes to move writing into a publishable form.

1. "Scholarship is based on community and conversation" (2002, p. 72).

   Work to situate your writing within the context of the existing conversations in the literature.

2. "Writing is a form of thinking, and thus a tool to use from the very beginning of a research project" (2002, p. 72).

   Writing is a continuous act that must evolve throughout a research project.

3. "It makes sense to seek advice throughout the writing process" (2002, p. 72).

   Many novice writers mistakenly think that publication is a solitary act rather than recognizing early on that the most successful writers are collaborating at all stages of research projects, including the writing up of the final research report and converting it into a publishable manuscript.

4. "Management is required" (2002, p. 73).

   Advanced planning and organizational skills are a must for bringing projects to fruition.

Huff's (1999) *Writing for Scholarly Publication* is an excellent resource for novice researchers interested in learning to convert their research into publications. Incorporating some of Huff's exercises into a qualitative research class can be a productive way of easing novice researchers forward into this type of writing.

Other highly practical and useful ideas can be culled from the work of active bloggers such as Pat Thomson (*https://patthomson.net*) and Raul Pacheco-Vega (*www.raulpacheco.org/blog*). Both are active on Twitter (@ThomsonPat and @raulpacheco, respectively), and you can find more about academic writing on Twitter by searching for the hashtag #Acwri (*https://twitter.com/Acwri*).

These are wonderful resource sites to include in weekly readings for novice researchers from any content or discipline and arranged in manageable bits to help students contemplate strategies and small-step actions.

O'Hara, Lower, and Mulvihill (in press) suggest the following common areas that deserve attention in the mentoring of novice researchers interested in learning how to publish:

1. What resources are available to students on-campus to help them make the best use of databases?

2. How do students develop both long-term and short-term publishing goals?

3. How do students learn academic writing?

4. How do students learn the time and task management skills needed to accomplish this type of writing?

5. What role do academic conferences play in the publishing process?

6. How do scholars select the most appropriate journal for their work?

7. What happens when a scholar receives a "revise and resubmit" decision from an editor?

8. How do scholars emotionally deal with rejection?

Given the finite period of time for a graduate research methods course, these eight areas might be useful to prioritize in order to keep this aspect of the course in the proper proportion.

In addition, we have found it very helpful to partner with others on campus to build the report-writing skills novice researchers need, such as reference librarians or information specialist librarians within university libraries (Bussell, Hagman, & Guder, 2017; Lindstrom & Shonrock, 2006; Phelps-Ward, Mulvihill, Jarrell, & Habich, 2015), campus writing center professionals, or panels of faculty and graduate students who have been successful at collaborating with each other for publication.

When students are connecting the outcomes of your course with the writing process for their research reports, such as doctoral dissertations, master's theses, and/or refereed journal articles, it may help to provide various ways for them to understand how each chapter or section of their writing has a particular job. For example, they may benefit by repeatedly hearing that the primary question to keep asking themselves while preparing section 4 or chapter 4 (i.e., data analysis) of their research report is "What does this mean?" Arranging and interpreting data in relation to the purpose of the study and the research questions, must arrive in section 4 or chapter 4 as a sophisticated piece of writing so there is a clear progression leading to a discernible argument.

Thinking about research while doing it is crucial for the development of the research and for the research to evolve. This type of research thinking is best guided by writing prompts and questions from instructors or mentors that help novice researchers learn the habits of mind required to seamlessly engage in various forms of reflexivity to help advance the project. Regularly reiterating to students the important connection between reading and writing can't be overemphasized. Building strategies and skills for *reading* qualitative research, with an eye toward methodologies and methods, along with a prose that easily moves a reader from one dimension of the writing to another, will help students build the *writing* skills they need to best communicate their projects. Likewise, the more time students spend working out the puzzles presented as they engage in the writing act, the more sophisticated readers of qualitative research they will become.

Writing Doctoral Dissertations, Master's Theses, and Refereed Journal Articles

While dissertations, research reports, master's theses, and articles for journals all have some elements in common, there are also differences in structuring them depending on the requirements from different institutions and journals. Dissertations and theses follow the five-chapter format with an occasional sixth chapter that has conclusions. The five sections or chapters are typically the introduction, the review of literature, methodology, findings, and discussion. At times, a chapter called conclusion is also added.

Teaching about the Different Sections through Examples

We typically give students an assignment where they choose an article or dissertation they are already reading for their own research and take it apart so that they can find out what the introduction does and what goes into the methods or findings. This process helps students to understand how the different sections of the article or dissertation work together. It also helps students to structure their own writing.

Low-Stakes Writing—or Practice Writing as a Pedagogical Strategy

We consider writing to be a way to clarify thinking, and as a result, we build writing into almost, if not all, class sessions in qualitative research. Teaching qualitative writing means emphasizing writing as part of the research process so that it is not seen as something to be put off until the inevitable moment arrives and then panic at what seems to be an insurmountable task—that of pulling together notes, interview data, and various thoughts and readings into a story. To avoid this possible anxiety situation, informal or low-stakes writing all along the research process makes it easier for students to practice writing what they really want to say through the data or what story they want most to tell. While we do not diminish the importance of formal, polished writing, we believe that the stepping stones to writing for publication or for writing qualitative research can start with short pieces in class. Low-stakes writing can be a pedagogical strategy that is easy to implement and yet can yield major results. Ungraded low-stakes writing can be short memos with prompts that go through the arc of the research process. They could be 100-word exercises; below is an A–Z of word exercises to be used in a qualitative research course:

Write 100 words on:

a. What do you like about your research idea?

b. Why do you think your participants are ideal for your study?

c. Why did you choose your site?

d. Why did you choose your study design?

e. Make two quick points about how race/class/gender/sexuality/ (dis)ability are connected to your research.

f. Who will your research benefit?

g. Who might be angry about your research?

h. Who will use your research?

i. Who might misuse your research?

j. Who are you in connection with your participants?

k. Why or how is your study different from other studies on this topic?

l. How would you have to alter your research design if you decide to conduct an ethnography/autoethnography/life history/case study/phenomenology/community-based participatory action research?

m. What are two main ideas that keep cropping up in your interviews?

n. How are the ideas in your data related to your research question?

o. Compose a blurb about your study.

p. Describe your study participants.

q. What are the three main findings in your study?

r. What do you think you will find when you conduct your research?

s. Describe your emotions right now.

t. Name three everyday objects you carry and what meaning they have to you.

u. How do the participants in your study relate to one another?

v. What are your thoughts on a documentary that you regard as a qualitative research exemplar?

w. Describe a qualitative study you just read.

x. What are two challenges that you are facing in the research process?

y. What two questions do you have right now that you want answered?

z. How did two researchers answer the questions you had about specific research processes?

Most writers subscribe to the theory that it is easier to rewrite then write and therefore advise that qualitative writing should start even before the research itself starts. Wolcott (1999) advocates starting with a description of the site or the purpose of the study, while others suggest a memo or a note to oneself outlining all the presumptions and assumptions one has about the project itself. "What I Think I Will Find" may be a good title for a memo that one can write before the start of fieldwork. These suggestions all provide potential starting points for faculty when contemplating designing writing exercises with particular goals in mind for the students in their course. A classroom exercise related to low-stakes writing can be a discussion on titles of dissertations and articles. Having a conversation with students on what they think the title of their dissertation would be is a good starting point to help them think about the main ideas in their research study.

"Workshopping" as a Method to Teach Writing Qualitative Research

In the spirit of writing "shitty first drafts," in the words of Lamott (2007), the workshopping method takes the messy draft to a level of polish that is deserving of peer scrutiny. In this sense, it forces students to write for presentation to others rather than writing for oneself. The distinction is important since writing for oneself—as in writing a journal—can be casual and meandering, and while the same may be true of writing for others', the writer is usually a little more attentive and conscious of being read by a peer. This distinction is meant to ensure that the writer is putting forth the effort while at the same time presenting to a community of fellow writers and peers whose purpose is to try to help the writer through questioning, clarification, or through pointing out what is missing. The feedback in workshopping is to allow for a focus on one another's writing with the goal of making the product clearer and better while learning to write.

Creating Peer Circles for Workshopping Writing

The workshop method for writing is to ask students to create peer circles, and if time permits, allow one class session for writing and feedback. This activity can also be adapted online since students can share their preliminary findings or a first draft of their writing and ask for feedback from their peers. This level of feedback prior to the second or final draft that comes to the faculty not only ensures that the quality of writing is likely to be much improved, it also allows multiple readers to give feedback on the writing. We have suggested that each person receive feedback from two others. This allows everyone to give and receive feedback.

Writing Findings in Qualitative Research

We decided to write a little here about writing findings in qualitative research since this is a point where students repeatedly struggle. Creative analytic processes should lead qualitative researchers to the point of identifying themes, figuring out subthemes, and finding exemplars from the data that serve as evidence for those themes. However, a question that is worth discussing in class is whether coding and analysis are also findings, or are findings in qualitative research something different?

Making Claims from Data

After the data are all coded and themes have been decided upon, the question of how to move from themes and codes to findings is somewhat puzzling to many students. After students have chosen their themes and their data to support their themes and codes, they then have to ask themselves four questions:

1. "What do I want to say about the findings and themes that I want people to know?"
2. "What are some takeaways from this research?"
3. "What insight can be gleaned from this particular set of participants at these sites about the phenomena that I have been examining?"
4. "What new insight or knowledge has been added through this research?"

Organization, *accuracy*, and *importance* are three key words that can help students think about telling the story from their data.

Typically, students want to say everything about the data that they have gathered and it is not unlike seeing a neighbor's vacation photographs. After 18 pictures of the seagull on the beach, one wants to know, Well, what else? or What is the story here? It is the same with qualitative research findings. When presenting findings, the researcher has to orchestrate the main findings and tell the story without digressing into lesser, although interesting, by-lanes.

Making Meaning from Data

One can find those "aha" moments when things come together or a sudden connection is perceived and new ideas come forth that enable us to understand or layer the meanings already made during preliminary analysis. Meaning making is possible when we are aware of our own theoretical framework and units of analysis.

Telling the Lesser Stories through Summaries

Not all the stories make up the major findings and yet it may be important to summarize or briefly mention those stories that are not necessarily followed up in the research. It may be important to tell the reader that those were stories that did not lend themselves to answering the research question chosen by the researcher.

Using Pseudonyms or Composites for People and Places in Qualitative Research Findings

What parts of the findings should be fictionalized or presented via pseudonyms? Recent advances in writing qualitative research have engaged fiction and different modes of fictionalization for a variety of purposes (Jones & Leavy, 2014; Leavy, 2012, 2016)—three of which have been identified in the literature as the most commonly used reasons for fictionalizing. The first is to further protect the participants by using composites to construct fictionalized characters from the data collected from several different people into one. This goes beyond the use of pseudonyms, which is the norm in most qualitative research, to help ensure confidentiality. However, this does not typically entail what might be referred to as fictionalizing. Students often ask about the difference between employing steps to help ensure confidentiality and making the data anonymous. They often conflate these two terms and need to be reminded to use the operationalized definitions offered by the IRB (which are guided by federal definitions of research). Similarly, students often have questions regarding the naming of research sites or other names of people or places that might be recognizable and by extension may compromise the confidentiality of the participants.

Writing the Discussion Chapter

The discussion chapter is the chapter or section that we like to refer to as "connecting the dots." This is the section where we suggest that students begin to think about how the findings relate to the literature, what the implications are of the study to the field and to practice, and how to help the reader see the bigger picture within which the study is located. We also suggest that students think about the new knowledge that their study is offering and reiterate in this section why it matters.

Acknowledge Limitations and Delimitations

Along with writing the discussion section, students need to learn to acknowledge the limitations of the study. Explaining to students that limitations are not problems and instead increase the strength and focus of the research conducted, helps them understand that research processes are continuous and that the process extends after their dissertation or article. This is also the place to refer to delimitations or the deliberate choices made by the researcher that set the boundaries of the study. It is also important that students understand the differences between limitations and delimitations.

Writing Articles during and after the Dissertation

Articles can be written from findings after the dissertation is completed. However, during the dissertation, those by-lanes that we referred to— the stories not told in the main findings—can come in useful in writing those shorter stories from the data. The data gathered will never go to waste and instead can be saved for writing articles over time.

Writing for Journals and Conferences

There are several venues where writing for journal articles has been tackled and it is not our intention to repeat those here (see, e.g., Hiemstra, 2001; Silvia, 2007). The most important point for students to understand is that when writing for a particular venue—be it journals for articles or book reviews—it is important to actually read the journal to understand the journal's scope. Reading examples will help students to write to the audience that the journal is directed toward. A practitioner journal is likely to have different criteria from a research journal. Our main advice to students around writing has been to read and practice and as a first draft, submit articles to conferences. Presenting at conferences gives students confidence and feedback that can lead them in the direction of publication. Practice with presentations can help students think through their study. (Exercise 10.2 on structuring practice presentations is offered later in this chapter.) In terms of journal submissions, we also caution students that submissions involve submitting, resubmitting, and dealing with rejections. Learning how to work with "revise and resubmits" is another topic that can be tackled if there is time in the course. It is our experience that since lack of sufficient time is a factor in qualitative courses, these topics are best addressed in the one-on-one mentoring sessions with doctoral students and their advisors. We also suggest developing a parallel set of activities in doctoral programs that focus on doctoral students' professional development where these questions and issues can be addressed.

What Is Quality in Qualitative Research?

An important part of learning qualitative research is to understand what represents quality in qualitative research. Looking at exemplars with a critical eye to learn from good examples and to be able to speculate what could have been done differently is part of the reflective thinking necessary for qualitative researchers. How can we teach students how to recognize high-quality work in qualitative research? How can we teach and learn to examine study findings and determine whether we got it right (Stake, 1995) and whether a researcher whose work we are reading got it right? Are the findings of value and substance? Applying quantitative criteria to qualitative studies has proved to be cumbersome, leading to the realization that qualitative studies need to develop criteria applicable to judging qualitative work. What types of questions and criteria should we hold up to qualitative research to determine the quality of a study? If the researcher is the instrument of the research, what types of criteria are appropriate to understand whether the researcher has conducted the study so that the study can be judged trustworthy? Within the qualitative research community, there are several viewpoints with regard to criteria for judging qualitative work. Hope and Waterman (2003) have summarized the positions taken by qualitative researchers on this issue. According to Hope and Waterman, one position is to apply criteria similar to quantitative research, a second is to advocate a different set of principles, and a third group of scholars question the appropriateness of any preset criteria and tend to reject them to judge quality in qualitative research.

The first group of scholars apply quantitative terminology to qualitative research (Field & Morse, 1985; Morse, Barrett, Mayan, Olson, & Spiers, 2002) and argue that there is nothing to be gained by using alternative terminology, "which on analysis, often prove to be identical to the traditional terms of reliability and validity" (Long & Johnson,

2000, p. 30). Morse et al. assert that if the researcher follows verification strategies, then validity and reliability, and thereby quality, will be achieved. LeCompte and Goetz (1982) similarly attempted to search for and find qualitative terms and ways to confirm and validate qualitative research in ways that paralleled quantitative research. They applied the issues of validity and reliability to qualitative research by examining selection, mortality, maturation, observer effects, and history, and studied the transferability of the study to other contexts. Some scholars within qualitative traditions argue that the terms *validity* and *reliability* are usually not used by qualitative researchers because of their association with quantitative research (Neuman, 2006). In addition, as Neuman points out, qualitative researchers tend to use and apply the terms in different ways.

Lincoln and Guba (1985) introduced the term *trustworthiness* as a way to explain the degree of rigor in qualitative research and proposed four criteria that would determine trustworthiness: credibility, transferability, dependability, and confirmability. Credibility can be seen in the degree to which the findings are congruent with reality. Transferability would require that sufficient details be provided to the reader of the study to determine whether the research findings can be applied to other contexts. Dependability would need a documentation of the research process by the researcher so that details of how data were gathered and what criteria were used for data collection and analysis are provided. Confirmability seeks to ensure that the findings of the study are the result of participants' perspectives and not a result of preferences on the part of the researcher. Confirmability can be arrived at through documentation of memos, details of participants' perspectives, raw data from transcripts, and field notes. While Guba and Lincoln (1989) have regarded member checks (the process of verifying data analysis with participants) or peer checking (a panel of experts examining the analysis to possibly arrive at similar analyses) as crucial for establishing credibility, other scholars (e.g., Sandelowski, 1993) have rejected these criteria arguing that if reality is multiple and constructed, we can hardly expect expert panels or participants to arrive at the same categories and themes as the researcher.

It is our stance that there are some quality indicators that are consistent across different types of qualitative studies. If we examine the different sets of criteria for quality proposed by scholars, we can discern some similar criteria across them. Creswell (2013) offered a short list of characteristics of a "good" qualitative study. They are formulated primarily around the process and procedures employed by researchers. They include rigorous data collection, framing the study within qualitative research principles and characteristics, and ensuring that a qualitative approach is used—that is, the researcher begins with a singular focus, the study includes detailed methods, the researcher analyzes data multiple times to reflect deeper levels of thinking, the researcher writes persuasively, the study reflects the cultural and personal experiences of the researcher, and the study is ethical. Similarly, Richardson (2000) suggested criteria for advocacy and participatory research—that is, substantive contribution, aesthetic merit, reflexivity, impact, and expression of reality. Charmaz (2006), in the same vein, suggests criteria to apply to grounded theory studies. She suggests that researchers ask themselves a series of questions that can evaluate the theory developed in the study—that is, questions on the completeness of the study, raising major categories, and increased scope and depth of analysis; strong theoretical links between categories; increased understanding of the phenomena; implications of the analysis for furthering understanding; and that the contribution and significance of the theory can be used to evaluate the study.

The different criteria developed by the various scholars all have features in common that we can find distilled into the comprehensive "eight big-tent criteria" by Tracy (2010), summarized as follows:

1. Worthy topic—topic is relevant, timely, and significant.

2. Rigor—the study shows sufficient data and time in the field, theoretical constructs are used, data collection and analyses processes are detailed and documented, and procedures used are appropriate for the study.

3. Sincerity—the study shows evidence of self-reflexivity regarding the values and assumptions of the researcher and transparency regarding the challenges of the research process. Sincerity is also characterized by an ethical stance toward the research and participants.

4. Credibility—thick description, crystallization, multivocality, and member reflections.

5. Resonance—research is presented and resonates with readers through aesthetics and presentation, naturalistic generalizations, and transferability or when readers feel that the story overlaps with their own life situations.

6. Significance—the research produces significant contributions conceptually, methodologically, and practically.

7. Ethical—the research is conducted ethically with attention to situational ethics, relational ethics, procedural ethics, and ethics for leaving or exiting the field.

8. Meaningful coherence—the study achieves what it starts out to do, and the procedures, literature, findings, and interpretations are all aligned and interconnected.

These criteria are flexible enough to be adapted to different studies. Quality in research is linked to the degree to which the research is construed as believable or the extent to which one can put one's trust in the findings or the methods of the research. Spillane and Miele (2007) point out that "research does not construct evidence, people do" (p. 47), thereby emphasizing that trustworthiness of research lies in the value of accepting the research findings as relevant to the purposes of the study. Knowledge production is scrutinized by the scholarly community. For students this community is often their professors, dissertation committee members, and peers, and as they proceed to participate as professionals in their jobs, they are then also subject to the scrutiny and dialogue within the professional community. Therefore, two sets of communities are likely to examine scholarship for its logic, procedures, ethics, and corresponding findings. The first is the community of practice (Lave & Wenger, 1991) and the second is the community of scholars.

Cassell, Bishop, Symon, Johnson, and Buehring (2009) argue that to learn to become effective qualitative researchers who are able to judge quality in research, we need to facilitate learning conditions so that we introduce students to three processes as researchers: reflection, reflexivity, and phronesis. Reflection is to critically reflect on readings and field work; reflexivity is the process by which students become aware of who they are, their assumptions, and preconceived ideas in relation to their study; and phronesis, often translated as practical wisdom, is the ability to discern or learn to reason about what needs to be done (Birmingham, 2004). In previous chapters, we discussed reflexivity in detail and how to teach the concept to students through a variety of activities. Here, we include Exercise 10.1 to bring students closer to learning to make decisions about their research even while they are engaged in it. To introduce students to a conversation with their peers on the quality of qualitative studies, we suggest the following activity.

Classroom Exercise 10.1. A Dialogue on Quality

GOAL: To get students to think about evaluative criteria of qualitative studies and discuss the evidence for each quality criterion.

OUTCOMES: Students learn to pay attention to some of the key features and characteristics of qualitative research and to formulate arguments advocating their perspective with evidence.

TIME: 30 minutes.

GUIDELINES FOR THE EDUCATOR: Divide the class into small groups and give an article to each group. You may decide to give a dissertation depending on how advanced the students are. Each group should read the article or dissertation ahead of time and come to class prepared to think about the different criteria for judging quality. Ask students to have a discussion in small groups comparing the big-tent criteria to the article or dissertation. Ask students to evaluate the article or dissertation against the criteria.

GUIDELINES TO SHARE WITH STUDENTS: Having read the dissertation or article, read the article by Tracy (2010) on the big-tent criteria for judging quality in qualitative research.

Tracy, S. J. (2010). Qualitative quality: Eight "big-tent" criteria for excellent qualitative research. *Qualitative Inquiry, 16*(10), 837–851.

In small groups, find the evidence for each of the quality indicators that Tracy (2010) has mentioned.

Reflect on the following questions and discuss in your small groups: What quality indicators were easy to find and which ones did you find challenging to locate? Are there other points or indicators that you found that should be included in the "big-tent" criteria? Explain those points to your peers.

Exercise 10.1 helps students to apply the criteria to studies and become familiar with the different procedures, assumptions, ethics, and the ways in which they can be reported in studies. The exercise can facilitate and deepen students' reflexive understanding of their data.

Exercise 10.2 can give students practice in presentation skills and in crafting a presentation for their dissertation defenses or for conference presentations. The exercise can also prepare students to present to a community of practice and a community of professionals.

Classroom Exercise 10.2. Presenting the Study in a Conference Format

GOAL: To create conditions for students to present their study to their peers and receive feedback; to create conditions where students can learn to apply quality criteria and defend their choices; and to help students learn to ask questions of their own and of a peer's study, with a view to strengthen it.

OUTCOMES: Students learn to practice presenting their study, defend choices they made, and learn to discuss their study in a formal format.

TIME: 1 hour and 15 minutes per panel of three or four students.

GUIDELINES FOR THE EDUCATOR: This activity can be adapted so that a poster session is organized instead of panel presentations. If possible, these presentations should be open to all graduate students and to faculty and similarly with the poster session, should that be opted for instead.

Ask students to prepare a 15-minute presentation of their study excerpted from their final papers for the course as they would for a conference. This helps students think about how to excerpt from longer papers and speak to an audience about their research. Keep a stack of index cards ready for the audience to offer feedback for presenters. Distribute the index cards to the audience and ask them to write the names of students on separate cards. Gather up the cards at the end of each presentation panel and offer them to the speakers to whom they pertain. Students need to think about the quality of qualitative research as they consider the writing and presentations of their peers. To do this, they need to keep in mind that qualitative research quality is determined in a number of ways, which they would have already discussed in class.

GUIDELINES TO SHARE WITH STUDENTS: Prepare a 15-minute presentation of your study that includes the reason for research, questions for research, methods, findings, and implications or significance of the research. Justify all the choices you have made by creating a narrative arc that flows from one section to another.

After you listen to each of your peers' presentations, note feedback for the speaker on an index card. Offer one positive comment and either one comment that can help the speaker improve his or her work or one question about his or her presentation.

This activity is useful to teach students how to take suggestions offered and rework their papers or think about how to go deeper in their analysis or convey their findings differently.

Pedagogically, one of the aims of all teachers is to scaffold researchers into independence and induct them into a community of scholars. Students in research methods courses at the end of the semester are usually ready to take the tentative steps to becoming part of a community of scholars and a community of practice. The activities in this chapter were designed to assist them in their growth and movement.

Teachers can use Table 10.1 to help increase the ways students can build the ability to conduct a self-analysis related to their own studies.

CHAPTER SUMMARY

In this chapter, we offered some ways that those teaching qualitative research can approach teaching students about writing qualitative research reports and manuscripts for publication. Pedagogical strategies of low-stakes writing, writing circles, or peer writing, and writing for journals and conferences have also been described. In addition, we discussed ways to think about quality in qualitative research and how to present to peers and participate in a scholarly community.

TABLE 10.1. Self-Analysis of Qualitative Study

1. Audit trail	Has the researcher given a sense of the detailed notes that he or she kept during the research?
2. Member checking	Has the researcher attempted to check back with participants regarding the accuracy of the data or findings?
3. Thick description	Has the researcher given enough detail that the qualitative descriptions are vivid?
4. Findings and sources of data	Do the findings emerge from the data cited?
5. Are the data sufficient?	This will be evident from the claims being made from the data. If there are not enough data, the claims will be weak and data saturation may not have been reached.
6. Are the data findings well organized?	Do they tell a story that is coherent?
7. Are the findings significant?	Do the findings tell us why the study is needed, addressing the "so what?" of the study?

Conclusion: Final Thoughts

Teaching is a learning activity and our endeavor in this book has been to share what we enjoy. Our own teaching journeys have been informed by a holistic pedagogy—one that is in a constant state of becoming and remains unfinished. Holistic pedagogy has no simple definition, easy-to-follow steps, or clear prescriptions. By holistic pedagogy we have meant a pedagogy that is attentive, curious, and imaginative, and takes into account the bodies and minds and spirits of those who walk into our classrooms and with whom we have the honor of interactions, conversations, and dialogue. We shared in this book what we learned from our experiences and through our dialogues with students, coresearchers, and co-learners. Our love for qualitative research and our conviction that it makes us more aware human beings leads us to think of it as a platform with transformative potential. We offer this book in the spirit that it be taken further, experimented with, and not looked upon as a prescription but rather as a catalyst for your own imaginative roads and your own voices. Our journey into pedagogies continues after this book and into our future projects.

References

Abboud, S., Kim, S. K., Jacoby, S., Mooney-Doyle, K., Waite, T., Froh, E., et al. (2017). Co-creation of a pedagogical space to support qualitative inquiry: An advanced qualitative collective. *Nurse Education Today, 50,* 8–11.

Agar, M. (1999). How to ask for a study in qualitatisch. *Qualitative Health Research, 9*(5), 684–697.

Agar, M. H. (2004). Know when to hold 'em, know when to fold 'em: Qualitative thinking outside the university. *Qualitative Health Research, 14*(1), 100–112.

Almond, P., & Apted, M. (Directors). (1964–present). *The UP series* [Motion picture on DVD]. United Kingdom: ITV Granada Television.

Anderson, E. (1978/1981). *A place on the corner.* Chicago: University of Chicago Press.

Baltar, F., & Brunet, I. (2012). Social research 2.0.: Virtual snowball sampling method using Facebook. *Internet Research, 22*(1), 57–74.

Banks, J. A. (1998). The lives and values of researchers: Implications for educating citizens in a multicultural society. *Educational Research, 27*(7), 4–17.

Bateson, G., & Mead, M. (1942). Balinese character: A photographic analysis. *New York Academy of Sciences, 2,* 17–92.

Becker, H. S. (2010). *Writing for social scientists: How to start and finish your thesis, book, or article.* Chicago: University of Chicago Press.

Belcher, W. L. (2009). Reflections on ten years of teaching writing for publication to graduate students and junior faculty. *Journal of Scholarly Publishing, 40*(2), 184–200.

Belcher, W. L. (n.d.). How to teach a journal article writing class. Retrieved from *www.wendybelcher.com/writing-advice/teach-journal-article-writing-class.*

Benton, A., Androff, D., Barr, B., & Taylor, S. (2011). Of quant jocks and qual outsiders: Doctoral student narratives on the quest for training in qualitative research. *Qualitative Social Work, 11,* 232–248.

Berg, B. L. (2009). Designing projects and concept mapping. In *Qualitative research methods for the social sciences* (7th ed., pp. 41–51). Boston: Allyn & Bacon.

Besen-Cassino, Y. (2014). *Consuming work: Youth labor in America.* Philadelphia: Temple University Press.

Bhattacharya, K. (2016). The vulnerable academic: Personal narratives and strategic de/colonizing of academic structures. *Qualitative Inquiry, 22*(5), 309–321.

Bhattacharya, K. (2017). *Fundamentals of qualitative research: A practical guide.* Abingdon, UK: Taylor & Francis.

Biggs, J. (1996). Enhancing teaching through constructive alignment. *Higher Education, 32*(3), 347–364.

Birks, M., Chapman, Y., & Francis, K. (2008). Memoing in qualitative research: Probing data and processes. *Journal of Research in Nursing, 13*(1), 68–75.

Birmingham, C. (2004). Phronesis: A model for pedagogical reflection. *Journal of Teacher Education, 55*(4), 313–324.

Blank, G. (2004). Teaching qualitative data analysis to graduate students. *Social Science Computer Review, 22,* 187–196.

Bloom, B. S. (Ed.). (1956). *Taxonomy of educational objectives: Vol. 1. Cognitive domain.* New York: McKay.

Bogdan, R. C., & Biklen, S. K. (2007). *Qualitative research for education: An introduction to theory and methods* (5th ed). Boston: Allyn & Bacon.

Boote, D. N., & Beile, P. (2005). Scholars before researchers: On the centrality of the dissertation literature review in research preparation. *Educational Researcher, 34*(6), 3–15.

Booth, A., Sutton, A., & Papaioannou, D. (2016). *Systematic approaches to a successful literature review.* London: SAGE.

Borgès Da Silva, R. (2013, September–October). Taxonomy and typology: Are they really synonymous? *Sante Publique, 25*(5), 633–637.

Bourdieu, P., & Wacquant, L. J. (1992). *An invitation to reflexive sociology.* Chicago: University of Chicago Press.

Breuer, F., & Schreier, M. (2007, January). Issues in learning about and teaching qualitative research methods and methodology in the social sciences. *Forum: Qualitative Social Research, 8*(1), Art 30.

Briney, K. (2015). *Data management for researchers: Organize, maintain, and share your data for research success.* Exeter, UK: Pelagic.

Brown, R. N. (2013). When black girls look at you: An anti-narrative photo-poem. In *Hear our truths: The creative potential of black girlhood* (pp. 98–138). Champaign: University of Illinois Press.

Burke, L. A., & Miller, M. K. (2001, May). Phone interviewing as a means of data collection: Lessons learned and practical recommendations. In *Forum: Qualitative Social Research, 2*(2), Art 7.

Bussell, H., Hagman, J., & Guder, C. S. (2017). Research needs and learning format preferences of graduate students at a large public university: An exploratory study. *College and Research Libraries, 78*(7), 978–998.

Cammarota, J., & Fine, M. (Eds.). (2008). Youth participatory action research: A pedagogy for transformational resistance. In *Revolutionizing education:*

Youth participatory action research in motion (pp. 1–11). New York: Routledge.

Carr, E. C. J., & Worth, A. (2001). The use of the telephone interview for research. *Nursing Times Research, 6,* 511–524.

Carspecken, P., & Apple, M. (1992). Critical qualitative research. In M. LeCompte, W. Millroy, & J. Preissley (Eds.), *Handbook of critical research in education* (pp. 507–554). San Diego, CA: Academic Press.

Carter, S., & Pitcher, R. (2010). Extended metaphors for pedagogy: Using sameness and difference. *Teaching in Higher Education, 15,* 579–589.

Casey, B. (2009). Arts-based inquiry in nursing education. *Contemporary Nurse, 32*(1–2), 69–82.

Cassell, C., Bishop, V., Symon, G., Johnson, P., & Buehring, A. (2009). Learning to be a qualitative management researcher. *Management Learning, 40*(5), 513–533.

Chambers, R. (1997). *Whose reality counts?: Putting the first last.* London: Intermediate Technology Development Group.

Charmaz, K. (1990). "Discovering" chronic illness: Using grounded theory. *Social Science and Medicine, 30*(11), 1161–1172.

Charmaz, K. (2001). Grounded theory. In R. M. Emerson (Ed.), *Contemporary field research: Perspectives and formulations* (pp. 335–352). Prospect Heights, IL: Waveland Press.

Charmaz, K. (2006). *Constructing grounded theory: A practical guide through qualitative research.* London: SAGE.

Charmaz, K. (2015). Teaching theory construction with initial grounded theory tools: A reflection on lessons and learning. *Qualitative Health Research, 25*(12), 1610–1622.

Chavez, C. (2008). Conceptualizing from the inside: Advantages, complications and demands on insider positionality. *The Qualitative Report, 13*(3), 474–494. Retrieved from *http://nsuworks.nova.edu/tqr/vol13/iss3/9.*

Chenail, R. J. (1997). Keeping things plumb in qualitative research. *The Qualitative Report, 3*(3), 1–8. Retrieved from *http://nsuworks.nova.edu/tqr/vol3/iss3/6.*

Chenail, R. J. (2011). Interviewing the investigator: Strategies for addressing instrumentation and researcher bias concerns in qualitative research. *The Qualitative Report, 16*(1), 255–262. Retrieved from *http://nsuworks.nova.edu/tqr/vol16/iss1/16.*

Clark, R., & Lang, A. (2002). Balancing yin and yang: Teaching and learning qualitative data analysis within an undergraduate quantitative data analysis course. *Teaching Sociology, 30*(3), 348–360.

Collier, D. R., Moffatt, L., & Perry, M. (2015). Talking, wrestling, and recycling: An investigation of three analytic approaches to qualitative data in education research. *Qualitative Research, 15*(3), 389–404.

Connell, J., Barkham, M., Cahill, J., Gilbody, S., & Madill, A. (2006). *A systematic scoping review of the research in higher and further education.* Lutterworth, UK: British Association for Counselling & Psychotherapy.

Cook, S. H., & Frances Gordon, M. (2004). Teaching qualitative research: A metaphorical approach. *Journal of Advanced Nursing, 47*(6), 649–655.

Creswell, J. W. (2003). *Research design: Qualitative, quantitative, and mixed method approaches* (2nd ed.). Thousand Oaks, CA: SAGE.

Creswell, J. W. (2013). *Qualitative inquiry and research design: Choosing among five approaches.* (3rd ed.). Thousand Oaks, CA: SAGE.

Creswell, J. W. (2018). *Research design: Qualitative, quantitative, and mixed methods approaches* (4th ed.). Thousand Oaks, CA: SAGE.

Cronin de Chavez, A., Backett-Milburn, K., Parry, O., & Platt, S. (2005). Understanding and researching wellbeing: Its usage in different disciplines and potential for health research and health promotion. *Health Education Journal, 64*(1), 70–87.

Crooks, V. A., Castleden, H., & Meerveld, I. T. V. (2010). Teaching research methods courses in human geography: Critical reflections. *Journal of Geography in Higher Education, 34*(2), 155–171.

Daly, J., & Lumley, J. (2002). Bias in qualitative research designs. *Australian and New Zealand Journal of Public Health, 26*(4), 299–300.

Davis, K., Drey, N., & Gould, D. (2009). What are scoping studies?: A review of the nursing literature. *International Journal of Nursing Studies, 46*(10), 1386–1400.

Deleuze, G., & Guattari, F. (1987). Introduction: Rhizome. In *A thousand plateaus: Capitalism and schizophrenia* (2nd ed., pp. 3–25). Minneapolis: University of Minnesota Press.

DeLyser, D. (2008). Teaching qualitative research. *Journal of Geography in Higher Education, 32*(2), 233–244.

DeLyser, D., Potter, A. E., Chaney, J., Crider, S., Debnam, I., Hanks, G., et al. (2013). Teaching qualitative research: Experiential learning in group-based interviews and coding assignments. *Journal of Geography, 112*(1), 18–28.

Denzin, N. K., & Giardina, M. D. (Eds.). (2011). *Qualitative inquiry and global crises.* Walnut Creek, CA: Left Coast Press.

Devault, M. (2010). From the seminar room. In W. Luttrell (Ed.), *Qualitative educational research: Readings in reflexive methodology and transformative practice* (pp.146–158). New York: Routledge.

Dewey, J. (1938). *Experience and education* (Kappa Delta Pi Lecture Series). Springfield, OH: Collier Books.

Drabble, L., Trocki, K. F., Salcedo, B., Walker, P. C., & Korcha, R. A. (2016). Conducting qualitative interviews by telephone: Lessons learned from a study of alcohol use among sexual minority and heterosexual women. *Qualitative Social Work, 15*(1), 118–133.

Drisko, J. W. (2016). Introducing a special issue: Teaching qualitative research and inquiry. *Qualitative Social Work, 15*(3), 303–306.

Duneier, M. (1999). *Sidewalk.* New York: Macmillan.

Dweck, C. (2006). *Mindset: The new psychology of success.* New York: Random House.

Earley, M. (2014). A synthesis of the literature on research methods education. *Teaching in Higher Education, 19,* 242–253.

Eco, U. (2015). *How to write a thesis.* Boston: MIT Press.

Eisenhart, M., & Jurow, A. S. (2011). Teaching qualitative research. In N. K. Denzin & Y. S. Lincoln (Eds.), *The SAGE handbook of qualitative research: Educational anthropology and research methodology* (pp. 699–714). Thousand Oaks, CA: SAGE.

Eisler, R. (2005). Tomorrow's children: Education for a partnership world. In J. Miller (Ed.), *Holistic learning and spirituality in education: Breaking new ground* (pp. 47–68). Albany: State University of New York Press.

Eisner, E. W. (1997). The promise and perils of alternative forms of data representation. *Educational Researcher, 26*(6), 4–10.

Ellis, C. (2004). *The ethnographic I: A methodological novel about autoethnography.* Walnut Creek, CA: Alta Mira Press.

Elton, L. (2001). Research and teaching: Conditions for a positive link. *Teaching in Higher Education, 6*(1), 43–56.

Emerson, R. M., Fretz, R. I., & Shaw, L. L. (1995). Processing fieldnotes: Coding and memoing. In *Writing ethnographic fieldnotes* (pp. 142–168). Chicago: University of Chicago Press.

Fasoli, L. (2003). Reading photographs of young children: Looking at practices. *Contemporary Issues in Early Childhood, 4*(1), 32–47.

Ferguson, A. A. (2001). *Bad boys: Public schools in the making of black masculinity.* Ann Arbor: University of Michigan Press.

Field, P. A., & Morse, J. A. (1985). *Nursing research: The application of qualitative research.* London: Croom Helm.

Fink, L. D. (2003). *Creating significant learning experiences: An integrated approach to designing college courses.* San Francisco: Jossey-Bass. Retrieved from *www.unl.edu/philosophy/[L._Dee_Fink]_Creating_Significant_Learning_Experi(BookZZ.org).pdf.*

Foucault, M., & Deleuze, G. (1977). Intellectuals and power. In M. Foucault & D. F. Bouchard (Ed.), *Language, counter-memory, practice: Selected essays and interviews* (pp. 205–217). Ithaca, NY: Cornell University Press.

Frei, J., Alvarez, S. E., & Alexander, M. B. (2010). Ways of seeing: Using the visual arts in nursing education. *Journal of Nursing Education, 49*(12), 672–676.

Freire, P. (1972). *Pedagogy of the oppressed* (M. B. Ramos, Trans.). New York: Herder & Herder.

Freire, P. (2000). *Pedagogy of freedom: Ethics, democracy and civic courage.* New York: Rowman & Littlefield.

Fry, H., Ketteridge, S., & Marshall, S. (2009). *A handbook for learning and teaching in higher education: Enhancing academic practice* (3rd ed.). London: Routledge.

Galletta, A., & Cross, W. E. (2013). The semi-structured interview as a repertoire of possibilities. In A. Galletta (Ed.), *Mastering the semi-structured interview and beyond: From research design to analysis and publication* (pp. 45–72). New York: NYU Press.

Gans, H. J. (1999). Participant observation in the era of "ethnography." *Journal of Contemporary Ethnography, 28*(5), 540–548.

Gauntlett, D. (2005). *Moving experiences: Media effects and beyond* (Vol. 13). Bloomington: Indiana University Press.

Geertz, C. (1973). *The interpretation of cultures: Selected essays.* New York: Basic Books.

Gentry, C. (2011). *Imagination, possibility and wide-awakeness.* Presented at the Maxine Greene Salon at the Creativity, Imagination and Innovation symposium. Retrieved from *http://artsandhumanities.pressible.org/christine_gentry/wide-awakeness-maxine-greene*.

Georgiou, D., & Carspecken, P. (2002). Critical ethnography and ecological psychology: Conceptual and empirical explorations of a synthesis. *Qualitative Inquiry, 8*(6), 688–706.

Gerstenblatt, P. (2013). Collage portraits as a method of analysis in qualitative research. *International Journal of Qualitative Methods, 12*(1), 294–309.

Gillies, V., & Robinson, Y. (2012). Developing creative research methods with challenging pupils. *International Journal of Social Research Methodology, 15*(2), 161–173.

Giroux, H. (1985). Intellectual labor and pedagogical work: Rethinking the role of the teacher as intellectual, part I. *Phenomenology and Pedagogy, 3*(1), 20–32.

Glaser, B., & Strauss, A. (1967). *The discovery of grounded theory*. New York: de Gruyter.

Glogowska, M., Young, P., & Lockyer, L. (2011). Propriety, process and purpose: Considerations of the use of the telephone interview method in an educational research study. *Higher Education, 62*(1), 17–26.

Goffman, E. (1959). *The presentation of self in everyday life*. Garden City, NY: Doubleday.

Gold, R. L. (1958). Roles in sociological field observations. *Social Forces, 36*(3), 217–223.

Gouldner, A. W. (1970). *Coming crisis of western sociology*. New York: Basic Books.

Graham, L., & Schuwerk, T. J. (2017). Teaching qualitative research methods using *Undercover Boss*. *Communication Teacher, 31*(1), 11–15.

Gray, D. (2013). *Doing research in the real world* (3rd ed.). Thousand Oaks, CA: SAGE.

Greene, M. (1978). Wide-awakeness and the moral life. In *Landscapes of learning* (pp. 42–52). New York: Teachers College Press.

Guba, E. G., & Lincoln, Y. S. (1989). *Fourth generation evaluation*. London: SAGE.

Guruge, S., Hynie, M., Shakya, Y., Akbari, A., Htoo, S., & Abiyo, S. (2015, August). Refugee youth and migration: Using arts-informed research to understand changes in their roles and responsibilities. *Forum: Qualitative Social Research, 16*(3), Art 15.

Hagey, R. S. (1997). The use and abuse of participatory action research. *Chronic Diseases in Canada, 18*(1), 1–4.

Hamer, B. (Writer/Director). (2003). *Kitchen stories* [Motion picture on DVD]. Sweden: Bulbul Films.

Hammersley, M. (2004). Teaching qualitative methodology: Craft, profession or bricolage. In C. Seale, G. Gobo, J. F. Gubrium, & D. Silverman (Eds.), *Qualitative research practice* (pp. 549–560). Thousand Oaks, CA: SAGE.

Hammersley, M. (2012, June). *Is it possible to teach social research methods well today?* Paper presented at HEA Social Sciences Teaching and Learning Summit: Teaching Research Methods, University of Warwick, Coventry, UK.

Hammersley, M., & Atkinson, P. (1993). *Ethnography: Principles in practice.* London: Routledge.

Hannes, K., & Parylo, O. (2014). Let's play it safe: Ethical considerations from participants in a photovoice research project. *International Journal of Qualitative Methods, 13*(1), 255–274.

Harper, D. (2002). Talking about pictures: A case for photo elicitation. *Visual Studies, 17*(1), 13–26.

Harrison, B. (2002). Photographic visions and narrative inquiry. *Narrative Inquiry, 12*(1), 87–111.

Hatch, J. A. (2002). *Doing qualitative research in education settings.* Albany: State University of New York Press.

Heckathorn, D. D. (2011). Comment: Snowball versus respondent-driven sampling. *Sociological Methodology, 41*(1), 355–366.

Hellawell, D. (2006). Inside–out: Analysis of the insider–outsider concept as a heuristic device to develop reflexivity in students doing qualitative research. *Teaching in Higher Education, 11*(4), 483–494.

Hiemstra, R. (2001). Uses and benefits of journal writing. *New Directions for Adult and Continuing Education, 90,* 19–26.

Hogan, L., Bengoechea, E. G., Salsberg, J., Jacobs, J., King, M., & Macaulay, A. C. (2014). Using a participatory approach to the development of a school-based physical activity policy in an indigenous community. *Journal of School Health, 84*(12), 786–792.

Hope, K. W., & Waterman, H. A. (2003). Praiseworthy pragmatism?: Validity and action research. *Journal of Advanced Nursing, 44*(2), 120–127.

hooks, b. (1994). *Teaching to transgress: Education as the practice of freedom.* London: Routledge.

Howard, C., & Brady, M. (2015). Teaching social research methods after the critical turn: Challenges and benefits of a constructivist pedagogy. *International Journal of Social Research Methodology, 18*(5), 511–525.

Hubbard, J. (2007). *Lives turned upside down: Homeless children in their own words and photographs.* New York: Aladdin.

Huff, A. S. (1999). *Writing for scholarly publication.* Thousand Oaks, CA: SAGE.

Huff, A. S. (2002). Learning to be a successful writer. In D. Partington (Ed.), *Essential skills for management research* (pp. 72–83). Thousand Oaks, CA: SAGE.

Hunter, A., Lusardi, P., Zucker, D., Jacelon, C., & Chandler, G. (2002). Making meaning: The creative component in qualitative research. *Qualitative Health Research, 12*(3), 388–398.

Hurworth, R. E. (2008). *Teaching qualitative research: Cases and issues.* Rotterdam, The Netherlands: Sense.

Irvine, A., Drew, P., & Sainsbury, R. (2013). "Am I not answering your questions properly?": Clarification, adequacy and responsiveness in semi-structured telephone and face-to-face interviews. *Qualitative Research, 13*(1), 87–106.

Jack, D. C. (1999). Ways of listening to depressed women in qualitative research: Interview techniques and analyses. *Canadian Psychology, 40*(2), 91–101.

Jackson, A. Y., & Mazzei, L. A. (2013). Plugging one text into another: Thinking with theory in qualitative research. *Qualitative Inquiry, 19*(4), 261–271.

Jhally, S. (Director), & Kilbourne, J. (Writer). (2010). *Killing us softly 4: Advertising's image of women* [Motion picture on DVD]. United States: Media Education Foundation.

Johnson, R. B., & Onwuegbuzie, A. J. (2004). Mixed methods research: A research paradigm whose time has come. *Educational Researcher, 33*(7), 14–26.

Jones, K., & Leavy, P. (2014). A conversation between Kip Jones and Patricia Leavy: Arts-based research, performative social science and working on the margins. *The Qualitative Report, 19*(19), 1–7.

Kain, E. L., Buchanan, E., & Mack, R. (2001). Institutional research as a context for teaching methodological skills. *Teaching Sociology, 29*(1), 9–22.

Kamberelis, G., & Dimitriadis, G. (2013). *Focus groups: From structured interviews to collective conversations.* London: Routledge.

Kamler, B., & Thomson, P. (2008). The failure of dissertation advice books: Toward alternative pedagogies for doctoral writing. *Educational Researcher, 37*(8), 507–514.

Katz, S. (2015). Qualitative-based methodology to teaching qualitative methodology in higher education. *International Journal of Teaching and Learning in Higher Education, 27*(3), 352–363.

Kaufman, P. (2013). Scribo ergo cogito: Reflexivity through writing. *Teaching Sociology, 41*(1), 70–81.

Kaun, A. (2010). Open-ended online diaries: Capturing life as it is narrated. *International Journal of Qualitative Methods, 9*(2), 133–148.

Kephart, T., & Berg, B. (2002, March). *Gang graffiti analysis: A methodological model for data collection.* Paper presented at the annual meeting of Academy of Criminal Justice Sciences, Anaheim, CA.

Kerr, K. (1990). *The bristling woods.* New York: Bantam Books.

Kilburn, D., Nind, M., & Wiles, R. (2014). Learning as researchers and teachers: The development of a pedagogical culture for social science research methods. *British Journal of Educational Studies, 62*(2), 191–207.

Kingwell, M. A. (1995). *A civil tongue.* Philadelphia: University of Pennsylvania Press.

Kolb, A. Y., & Kolb, D. A. (2012). Experiential learning theory. In N. M. Seel (Ed.), *Encyclopedia of the sciences of learning* (pp. 1215–1219). New York: Springer.

Koro-Ljungberg, M. (2016). *Reconceptualizing qualitative research methodologies without methodology.* Thousand Oaks, CA: SAGE.

Koro-Ljungberg, M., Yendol-Hoppey, D., Smith, J. J., & Hayes, S. B. (2009). (E)pistemological awareness, instantiation of methods, and uninformed methodological ambiguity in qualitative research projects. *Educational Researcher, 38*(9), 687–699.

Korthagen, F. A. J. (2004). In search of the essence of a good teacher: Towards a more holistic approach in teacher education. *Teaching and Teacher Education, 20,* 77–97.

Kreber, C., Castleden, H., Erfani, N., & Wright, T. (2005). Self-regulated learning about university teaching: An exploratory study. *Teaching in Higher Education, 10*(1), 75–97.

Krueger, R. A. (1988). *Focus groups: A practical guide for applied research.* London: SAGE.

Krueger, R. A. (1994). *Focus groups: A practical guide for applied research* (2nd ed.). Thousand Oaks, CA: SAGE.

Kuhn, P. (2003, January). Thematic drawing and focused, episodic interview upon the drawing—a method in order to approach to the children's point of view on movement, play and sports at school. *Forum: Qualitative Social Research, 4*(1), Art 8.

Kusenbach, M. (2003). Street phenomenology: The go-along as ethnographic research tool. *Ethnography, 4*(3), 455–485.

Kvale, S. (1996). *Interviews. An introduction to qualitative research writing.* Thousand Oaks, CA: SAGE.

Ladson-Billings, G., & Tate, W. F. (Eds.). (2006). *Education research in the public interest: Social justice, action, and policy.* New York: Teachers College Press.

Lakoff, G., & Johnson, M. (1980). *Metaphors we live by.* Chicago: University of Chicago Press.

Lamott, A. (2007). *Bird by bird: Some instructions on writing and life.* New York: Anchor.

Lapum, J., & Hume, S. (2015). Teaching qualitative research: Fostering student curiosity through an arts-informed pedagogy. *The Qualitative Report, 20*(8), 1221–1233.

Lather, P. (2006). Paradigm proliferation as a good thing to think with: Teaching research in education as a wild profusion. *International Journal of Qualitative Studies in Education, 19*(1), 35–57.

Lather, P. (2012). *Getting lost: Feminist efforts toward a double(d) science.* Albany: State University of New York Press.

Lave, J., & Wenger, E. (1991). *Situated learning: Legitimate peripheral participation.* Cambridge, UK: Cambridge University Press.

Leavy, P. (2012). Fiction and the feminist academic novel. *Qualitative Inquiry, 18*(6), 516–522.

Leavy, P. (2016). *Fiction as research practice: Short stories, novellas, and novels.* New York: Routledge.

Leavy, P. (2017). *Research design: Quantitative, qualitative, mixed methods, arts-based, and community-based participatory research approaches.* New York: Guilford Press.

LeCompte, M. D., & Goetz, J. P. (1982). Problems of reliability and validity in ethnographic research. *Review of Educational Research, 52*(1), 31–60.

Lewis, A. E. (2003). *Race in the schoolyard: Negotiating the color line in classrooms and communities.* New Brunswick, NJ: Rutgers University Press.

Lewthwaite, S., & Nind, M. (2016). Teaching research methods in the social sciences: Expert perspectives on pedagogy and practice. *British Journal of Educational Studies, 64*(4), 413–430.

Li, S., & Seale, C. (2007). Learning to do qualitative data analysis: An observational study of doctoral work. *Qualitative Health Research, 17*(10), 1442–1452.

Lincoln, Y. S., & Guba, E. G. (1985). *Naturalistic inquiry* (Vol. 75). London: SAGE.

Lindstrom, J., & Shonrock, D. D. (2006). Faculty–librarian collaboration to achieve integration of information literacy. *Reference and User Services Quarterly, 46,* 18–23.

Lofland, J., & Lofland, L. H. (1995). Strategy five: Diagramming/typologizing/matrix making/concept charting/flow charting. In *Analyzing social settings: A guide to qualitative observation and analysis* (pp. 212–219). Belmont, CA: Wadsworth.

Loftsdóttir, K. (2002). Never forgetting?: Gender and racial-ethnic identity during fieldwork. *Social Anthropology, 10*(3), 303–317.

Long, T., & Johnson, M. (2000). Rigour, reliability and validity research. *Clinical Effectiveness in Nursing, 4*(1), 30–37.

Lorenz, W. (2003). European experiences in teaching social work research. *Social Work Education, 22*(1), 7–18.

Loxley, A., & Seery, A. (2008). Some philosophical and other related issues in insider research. In P. Sikes & A. Potts (Eds.), *Researching education from the inside: Investigations from within* (pp. 15–32). London: Routledge.

Luttrell, W. (2000, December). "Good enough" methods for ethnographic research. *Harvard Educational Review, 70*(4), 499–523.

Luttrell, W. (2010). *Qualitative educational research: Readings in reflexive methodology and transformative practice.* New York: Routledge.

Madriz, E. I. (1997). Images of criminals and victims: A study on women's fear and social control. *Gender and Society, 11*(3), 342–356.

Mann, C., & Stewart, F. (2000). *Internet communication and qualitative research: A handbook for researching online.* London: SAGE.

Marzano, R. J., & Kendall, J. S. (Eds.). (2006). *The new taxonomy of educational objectives.* Thousand Oaks, CA: Corwin Press.

Maxwell, J. A. (2008). Designing a qualitative study. In L. Bickman & D. J. Rog (Eds.), *The SAGE handbook of applied social research methods* (2nd ed., pp. 214–253). Thousand Oaks, CA: SAGE.

McKeachie, W., & Svinicki, M. (2013). *McKeachie's teaching tips.* Belmont, CA: Cengage Learning.

McNicoll, P. (2014). Issues in teaching participatory action research. *Journal of Social Work Education, 35*(1), 51–62.

Meier, D. (2002). *The power of their ideas: Lessons for America from a small school in Harlem.* Boston: Beacon Press.

Merton, R. (1972). Insiders and outsiders: A chapter in the sociology of knowledge. *American Journal of Sociology, 78*(1), 9–47.

Metz, M. H. (2001). Intellectual border crossing in graduate education: A report from the field. *Educational Researcher, 30*(5), 1–7.

Mezirow, J. (2003). Transformative learning as discourse. *Journal of Transformative Education, 1*(1), 58–63.

Miles, M., & Huberman, M. (1994). *Qualitative data analysis: An expanded sourcebook* (2nd ed.). Thousand Oaks, CA: SAGE.

Miller, G., & Happell, B. (2006). Talking about hope: The use of participant photography. *Issues in Mental Health Nursing, 27*(10), 1051–1065.

Miller, J. P. (2000). *Education and the soul: Toward a spiritual curriculum.* Albany: State University of New York Press.

Miller, J. (2005). *Holistic learning and spirituality in education.* Albany: State University of New York Press.

Mishler, E. G. (1991). *Research interviewing.* Boston: Harvard University Press.

Morris, E. (2011). *Believing is seeing: On the mysteries of photography.* London: Penguin Press.

Morse, J. M. (Ed.). (1994). *Critical issues in qualitative research methods.* Thousand Oaks, CA: SAGE.

Morse, J. (2003). Biasphobia. *Qualitative Health Research, 13*(7), 891–892.

Morse, J. (2004). Constructing qualitatively derived theory: Concept construction and concept typologies. *Qualitative Health Research, 14,* 1387–1395.

Morse, J. (2011). Molding qualitative health research. *Qualitative Health Research, 21,* 1019–1021.

Morse, J. M., Barrett, M., Mayan, M., Olson, K., & Spiers, J. (2002). Verification strategies for establishing reliability and validity in qualitative research. *International Journal of Qualitative Methods, 1*(2), 1–19.

Mulvihill, T. (2013). Mentoring, talking sticks, and academic spiritwalking. *The Learning Teacher Magazine, 4,* p. 12. Retrieved from *www.learning-teacher.eu/sites/learningteacher.eu/files/flipbook/421/Web/index.html.*

Mulvihill, T., & Swaminathan, R. (2012a). Creative qualitative inquiry: Innovative graduate level pedagogies shaped by educational technologies. *Journal of Educational Technology, 8*(3), 21–26.

Mulvihill, T. M., & Swaminathan, R. (2012b). Nurturing the imagination: Creativity processes and innovative qualitative research projects. *Journal of Educational Psychology, 5*(4), 1–8.

Mulvihill, T. M., & Swaminathan, R. (2013). Creativity and learning in the virtual sphere: Perspectives from doctoral students [Special issue]. *Journal of Educational Technology, 9*(3), 41–48.

Mulvihill, T. M., & Swaminathan, R. (2017). *Critical approaches to life writing methods in qualitative research.* New York: Routledge.

Mulvihill, T. M., & Swaminathan, R. (2019). *Secondary data analysis in qualitative research.* Manuscript under review.

Mulvihill, T. M., Swaminathan, R., & Bailey, L. C. (2015). Catching the "tail/tale" of teaching qualitative inquiry to novice researchers. *The Qualitative Report, 20*(9), 1490–1498. Retrieved from *http://nsuworks.nova.edu/tqr/vol20/iss9/13.*

Nakagawa, Y. (2000). *Education for awakening: An Eastern approach to holistic education.* Brandon, VT: Resource Center for Redesigning Education.

Naples, N. A. (2003). *Feminism and method: Ethnography, discourse analysis, and activist research.* New York: Routledge.

Nathan, R. (2006). *My freshman year: What a professor learned by becoming a student.* London: Penguin.

Neuman, W. L. (2006). *Social research methods: Qualitative and quantitative approaches.* Boston: Pearson.

Nichols, J. (2000). *The Milagro beanfield war: A novel* (Vol. 1). New York: Macmillan.

Nind, M., Kilburn, D., & Luff, R. (2015). The teaching and learning of social research methods: Developments in pedagogical knowledge [Editorial]. *International Journal of Social Research Methodology, 18*(5), 455–461.

Norton, L. (2009). Assessing student learning. In H. Fry, S. Ketteridge, & S. Marshall (Eds.), *Handbook for teaching and learning in higher education: Enhancing academic practice* (pp. 132–149). New York: Routledge.

O'Connor, D. L., & O'Neill, B. J. (2004). Toward social justice: Teaching qualitative research. *Journal of Teaching in Social Work, 24*(3–4), 19–33.

O'Hara, L., Lower, L., & Mulvihill, T. (in press). Mentoring graduate students in the publishing process: Methods to make it manageable and meaningful. *International Journal of Teaching and Learning in Higher Education.*

Opdenakker, R. (2006, September). Advantages and disadvantages of four interview techniques in qualitative research. *Forum: Qualitative Social Research, 7*(4), Art 11.

Palmer, P. J. (2010). *The courage to teach: Exploring the inner landscape of a teacher's life.* Edison, NJ: Wiley.

Panitz, T., & Panitz, P. (1998). Encouraging the use of collaborative learning in higher education. In J. J. F. Forest (Ed.), *University teaching: International perspectives* (pp. 161–201). New York: Garland.

Patel, N. V. (2003). A holistic approach to learning and teaching interaction: Factors in the development of critical learners. *International Journal of Educational Management, 17*(6), 272–284.

Patton, M. Q. (2016). *Qualitative research and evaluation methods.* London: SAGE.

Phelps-Ward, R., Mulvihill, T., Jarrell, L., & Habich, B. Y. (2015). Online distance education and embedded librarianship integration. In M. Khosrow-Pour (Ed.), *Encyclopedia of information science and technology* (3rd ed., pp. 2249–2257). Hershey, PA: IGI Global.

Phillips, D. C. (2006). A guide for the perplexed: Scientific educational research, methodolatry, and the gold versus platinum standards. *Educational Research Review, 1*(1), 15–26.

Pickles, D., King, L., & Belan, I. (2009). Attitudes of nursing students towards caring for people with HIV/AIDS: Thematic literature review. *Journal of Advanced Nursing, 65*(11), 2262–2273.

Polkinghorne, D. E. (2006). An agenda for the second generation of qualitative studies. *International Journal of Qualitative Studies on Health and Well-Being, 1*(2), 68–77.

Powdermaker, H. (1966). *Stranger and friend: The way of an anthropologist.* New York: Norton.

Preissle, J., & deMarrais, K. D. (2011). Teaching qualitative research responsively. In N. K. Denzin & M. D. Giardina (Eds.), *Qualitative inquiry and global crises* (pp. 13–39). Walnut Creek, CA: Left Coast Press.

Preissle, J., & Roulston, K. (2009). Trends and issues in teaching qualitative research. In M. Garner, C. Wagner, & B. Kawulich (Eds.), *Teaching research methods in the social sciences* (pp. 13–21). London: Ashgate.

Raddon, M., Raby, R., & Sharpe, E. (2009). The challenges of teaching qualitative coding: Can a learning object help? *International Journal of Teaching and Learning in Higher Education, 21,* 336–350.

Raingruber, B. (2009). Assigning poetry reading as a way of introducing students to qualitative data analysis. *Journal of Advanced Nursing, 65*(8), 1753–1761.

Rathwell, K., & Armitage, D. (2016). Art and artistic processes bridge knowledge systems about social–ecological change: An empirical examination with Inuit artists from Nunavut, Canada. *Ecology and Society, 21*(2), 21.

Redford, R. (Director), & Nichols, J. (Writer). (1988). *The Milagro beanfield war* [Motion picture on DVD]. United States: Universal.

Richardson, L. (2000). New writing practices in qualitative research. *Sociology of Sport Journal, 17*(1), 5–20.

Richardson, L., & St. Pierre, E. A. (2005). Writing: A method of inquiry. In N. K. Denzin & Y. S. Lincoln (Eds.), *The SAGE handbook of qualitative research* (3rd ed., pp. 959–978). Thousand Oaks, CA: SAGE.

Rinaldi, C. (2006). *In dialogue with Reggio Emilia: Listening, researching and learning.* London: Routledge Psychology Press.

Rom, M. C. (2015). Numbers, pictures, and politics: Teaching research methods through data visualizations. *Journal of Political Science Education, 11*(1), 11–27.

Rosenshine, B., & Meister, C. (1994). Reciprocal teaching: A review of the research. *Review of Educational Research, 64*(4), 479–530.

Rubin, H. J., & Rubin, I. S. (2011). *Qualitative interviewing: The art of hearing data* (3rd ed.). Thousand Oaks, CA: SAGE.

Sade-Beck, L. (2004). Internet ethnography: Online and offline. *International Journal of Qualitative Methods, 3*(2), 45–51.

Saldana, J. (2015). *The coding manual for qualitative researchers.* Los Angeles: SAGE.

Sandelowski, M. (1993). Rigor or rigor mortis: The problem of rigor in qualitative research revisited. *Advances in Nursing Science, 16*(2), 1–8.

Sargeant, S. (2012). "I don't get it": A critical reflection on conceptual and practical challenges in teaching qualitative methods. *Psychology Learning and Teaching, 11*(1), 39–45.

Sargent, J. (Director). (1997). *Miss Evers' boys* [Motion picture on DVD]. United States: HBO.

Saura, D. M., & Balsas, P. R. (2014). Interviewing and surveying over the phone: A reflexive account of a research on parenting. *Quality and Quantity, 48*(5), 2615–2630.

Schön, D. A. (1987). *Educating the reflective practitioner: Toward a new design for teaching and learning in the professions.* San Francisco, CA: Jossey-Bass.

Schratz, M., Walker, R., & Wiedel, J. (1995). Being there: Using pictures to see the invisible. In M. Schratz & R. Walker (Eds.), *Research as social change: New opportunities for qualitative research* (pp. 65–90). London: Routledge.

Seidman, I. (2005). Analyzing, interpreting, and sharing interview material. In *Interviewing as qualitative research: A guide for researchers in education and the social services* (3rd ed., pp. 115–138). New York: Teachers College Press.

Shon, P. C. H. (2015). *How to read journal articles in the social sciences: A very practical guide for students*. Thousand Oaks, CA: SAGE.

Silverman, D. (2011). *Interpreting qualitative data: A guide to the principles of qualitative research*. London: SAGE.

Silvia, P. J. (2007). *How to write a lot: A practical guide to productive academic writing*. Washington, DC: American Psychological Association.

Simons, M., & Elen, J. (2007). The "research–teaching nexus" and "education through research": An exploration of ambivalences. *Studies in Higher Education, 32*(5), 617–631.

Singh, A. A., & Lukkarila, L. (2017). *Successful academic writing: A complete guide for social and behavioral scientists*. New York: Guilford Press.

Smith, E. M. (2005). Telephone interviewing in healthcare research: A summary of the evidence. *Nurse Researcher, 12*(3), 32–41.

Smith, S. J. (1988). Constructing local knowledge: The analysis of self in everyday life. In J. Eyles & D. Smith (Eds.), *Qualitative methods in human geography* (pp. 17–38). Cambridge, UK: Polity Press.

Snowden, D. (Producer). (2011). Cynefin framework introduction. Retrieved from *http://cognitive-edge.com/videos/cynefin-framework-introduction*.

Somerville, M. (2013). *Water in a dry land: Place-learning through art and story*. London: Routledge.

Sommers, R. C. (1997). The quilting bee: A research metaphor. *The Qualitative Report, 3*(4), 1–3.

Sousa, D. A. (2011). *How the brain learns*. Thousand Oaks, CA: Corwin Press.

Spalter-Roth, R., & Van Vooren, N. (2008). What are they doing with a bachelor's degree in sociology?: Data brief on current jobs. *American Sociological Association*. Retrieved from *www.asanet.org/research-and-publications/research-sociology/research-briefs/what-are-they-doing-bachelors-degree-sociology-data-brief-current-jobs*.

Spillane, J. P., & Miele, D. B. (2007). Evidence in practice: A framing of the terrain. *Yearbook of the National Society for the Study of Education, 106*(1), 46–73.

Spradley, J. P. (1987). *The ethnographic interview*. New York: Holt, Rinehart and Winston.

Spronken-Smith, R. (2005). Implementing a problem-based learning approach for teaching research methods in geography. *Journal of Geography in Higher Education, 29*(2), 203–221.

St. Pierre, E. A. (2015). Practices for the "new" in the new empiricisms, the new materialisms, and post qualitative inquiry. In N. K. Denzin & M. D. Giardina (Eds.), *Qualitative inquiry and the politics of research* (pp. 75–95). Walnut Creek, CA: Left Coast Press.

St. Pierre, E. A. (2017). Post qualitative inquiry. In N. Denzin & M. Giardina (Eds.), *Qualitative inquiry in neoliberal times* (pp. 37–47). New York: Routledge.

Stake, R. E. (1995). *The art of case study research*. Thousand Oaks, CA: SAGE.

Steinberg, S., & Cannella, G. (Eds.). (2012). *Critical qualitative research reader*. New York: Lang.

Sternberg, R. J. (1989). Review of educating reason: Rationality, critical thinking, and education. *Analytic Teaching, 10,* 120–121.

Sudweeks, F., & Simoff, S. J. (1999). Complementary explorative data analysis: The reconciliation of quantitative and qualitative principles. In S. Jones (Ed.), *Doing Internet research: Critical issues and methods for examining the Net* (pp. 29–55). Thousand Oaks, CA: SAGE.

Swadener, B. B. (2005). Kenyan street children speak through their art. In L. D. Soto & B. B. Swadener (Eds.), *Power and voice in research with children* (pp. 137–149). New York: Lang.

Swaminathan, R. (1997). *"The charming sideshow": Cheerleading, girls' culture and schooling.* Unpublished doctoral dissertation, Syracuse University, NY.

Swaminathan, R., & Mulvihill, T. M. (2017). *Critical approaches to questions in qualitative research.* London: Routledge Press.

Sword, H. (2012). *Stylish academic writing.* Cambridge, MA: Harvard University Press.

Sword, H. (2017). *Air and light and time and space: How successful academics write.* Cambridge, MA: Harvard University Press.

Tavory, I., & Timmermans, S. (2014). *Abductive analysis: Theorizing qualitative research.* Chicago: University of Chicago Press.

Taylor, J. (2011). The intimate insider: Negotiating the ethics of friendship when doing insider research. *Qualitative Research, 11*(1), 3–22.

Tesch, R. (1990). *Qualitative analysis: Analysis types and software tools.* London: Falmer Press.

Tracy, S. J. (2010). Qualitative quality: Eight "big-tent" criteria for excellent qualitative research. *Qualitative Inquiry, 16*(10), 837–851.

Trier-Bieniek, A. (2012). Framing the telephone interview as a participant-centered tool for qualitative research: A methodological discussion. *Qualitative Research, 12*(6), 630–644.

Tuckman, B. W., & Jensen, M. A. C. (1977). Stages of small-group development revisited. *Group and Organization Studies, 2*(4), 419–427.

Tunnell, K. D. (2012). Reflections on visual field research. *International Journal of Qualitative Methods, 11*(4), 340–351.

Turney, L., & Pocknee, C. (2005). Virtual focus groups: New frontiers in research. *International Institute for Qualitative Methods, 4*(2), 32–43.

Twine, F. W. (2016). Visual sociology in a discipline of words: Racial literacy, visual literacy and qualitative research methods. *Sociology, 50*(5), 967–974.

Van Maanen, J. (2011). *Tales of the field: On writing ethnography.* Chicago: University of Chicago Press.

Vaughan, K. (2005). Pieced together: Collage as an artist's method for interdisciplinary research. *International Journal of Qualitative Methods, 4*(1), 27–52.

Venkatesh, S. A. (2008). *Gang leader for a day: A rogue sociologist takes to the streets.* London: Penguin.

Vygotsky, L. S. (1978). *Mind in society: The development of higher mental process.* Boston: Harvard University Press.

Wagner, C., Garner, M., & Kawulich, B. (2011). The state of the art of teaching research methods in the social sciences: Towards a pedagogical culture. *Studies in Higher Education, 36*(1), 75–88.

Waite, D. (2014). Teaching the unteachable: Some issues of qualitative research pedagogy. *Qualitative Inquiry, 20*(3), 267–281.

Wallace, M., & Wray, A. (2016). *Critical reading and writing for postgraduates.* Thousand Oaks, CA: SAGE.

Wang, C. C. (1999). Photovoice: A participatory action research strategy applied to women's health. *Journal of Women's Health, 8*(2), 185–192.

Wang, C., & Burris, M. A. (1997). Photovoice: Concept, methodology, and use for participatory needs assessment. *Health Education and Behavior, 24*(3), 369–387.

Wang, C., Burris, M. A., & Ping, X. Y. (1996). Chinese village women as visual anthropologists: A participatory approach to reaching policymakers. *Social Science and Medicine, 42*(10), 1391–1400.

Ward, V., House, A., & Hamer, S. (2009). Developing a framework for transferring knowledge into action: A thematic analysis of the literature. *Journal of Health Services Research and Policy, 14*(3), 156–164.

Welch, R. V., & Panelli, R. (2003). Teaching research methodology to geography undergraduates: Rationale and practice in a human geography programme. *Journal of Geography in Higher Education, 27*(3), 255–277.

Williams, J. (2010). Taking on the role of questioner: Revisiting reciprocal teaching. *The Reading Teacher, 64*(4), 278–281.

Wiseman, F. (Director/Producer/Writer). (1994). *High school II* [Motion picture on DVD]. United States: Zipporah Films.

Wolcott, H. F. (1999). *Ethnography: A way of seeing.* Lanham, MD: Altamira Press.

Wolcott, H. F. (2001). *Writing up qualitative research.* Newbury Park, CA: SAGE.

Wolcott, H. F. (2002). Writing up qualitative research . . . better. *Qualitative Health Research, 12*(1), 91–103.

Wolcott, H. F. (2009). *Writing up qualitative research* (3rd ed.). Thousand Oaks, CA: SAGE.

Wong, S., & Sumsion, J. (2013). Integrated early years services: A thematic literature review. *Early Years, 33*(4), 341–353.

Woodgate, R. L., Zurba, M., & Tennent, P. (2017). Worth a thousand words?: Advantages, challenges and opportunities in working with photovoice as a qualitative research method with youth and their families. *Forum: Qualitative Social Research, 18*(1), Art 2. Retrieved from *www.qualitative-research.net/index.php/fqs/article/view/2659.*

Woodley, X., & Lockard, M. (2016). Womanism and snowball sampling: Engaging marginalized populations in holistic research. *The Qualitative Report, 21*(2), 321–329.

Zinsser, W. (1983). *On writing well* (2nd ed.). New York: Harper & Row.

Zinsser, W. (2012). *On writing well* (30th anniv. ed.). New York: Harper & Row.

Index

Note. *f* or *t* following a page number indicates a figure or a table.

About the Authors

Raji Swaminathan, PhD, is Associate Professor in the Department of Educational Policy and Community Studies in the School of Education at the University of Wisconsin–Milwaukee. She has served as Director of Doctoral Studies and Chair of the Department and is a recipient of the university's Faculty Teaching Award. Dr. Swaminathan has authored or edited three previous books—two on qualitative research methods and one on the narratives of immigrant women. She is interested in and works in the areas of qualitative research, youth resilience, urban and alternative schools, creative pedagogies, and school leadership within qualitative research.

Thalia M. Mulvihill, PhD, is Professor of Higher Education and Social Foundations and Acting Assistant Provost at Ball State University. She has served as Director of two doctoral programs, as well as Director of the Certificate Program in Qualitative Research and Education and the Certificate Program in College and University Teaching. Dr. Mulvihill is coeditor of *The Teacher Educator* and author of four previous books related to qualitative research and innovative pedagogies. A recipient of numerous teaching, research, and mentoring awards, she is engaged in the study of historical and sociological issues in the fields of higher education, innovative pedagogies, educational leadership, and qualitative inquiry.